What Others Are Saying About This Book

"You bought this book because you or your loved ones are scared you may be killed by cancer. This book is a lifesaver for curing cancer. Dr. Loudon has put his heart into it, so to speak, based on his considerable medical experience. Follow the advice here, and you will be safer than any other method offered to you."

—by Professor Andrew Hague, Cell Sonic Corporation

Critical Non Invasive Treatment to Cure Grade III and IV Cancer

PLUS: PREVENTIVE CANCER PROCEDURES

DR. MERLE LOUDON

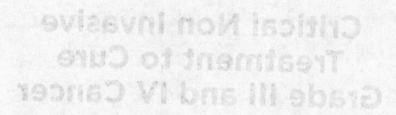

Critical Non-Invasive Treatment to Heal Grade III and IV Cancer
First edition, published 2021

By Dr. Merle Loudon
Cover design by Reprospace.com

The information in this book is to be used for informational use only. No words, sentences, paragraphs, foods, supplements, dosages, treatments, medications, advice, and procedures should be used without your physician's approval. The author has not intended for this book to be used as a cure, procedure, medication, or advice without a licensed medical professional and/or physician's consent. Although the author has made every attempt and effort to insure that the information in this book is correct, time, alternate procedures, new information, and new methods of treatments may change from the contents of this book. It has been written for educational and informational purposes only.

Published by Dr. Merle Loudon Publishing

Dedication

This book is dedicated to my wonderful wife, Sylvia. She has been very cooperative while I have sequestered myself in the computer room. She has gone through two cancer surgeries, two artificial knee joint surgeries, two artificial hip joints, (one twice), a fourteen-inch plate in her lower left femur, and two screws and a plate in her lower back. On August 2, 2020, Sylvia suffered a mild stroke. After 33 days of hospital and rehabilitation, she is in a wheelchair and can walk with help. Through it all, I admire her attitude and love of life. If she had a better diet in her younger years, I wonder if she would have had all of the problems and surgeries. She is a wonderful, caring wife.

I also want to dedicate my book to my wonderful daughter, Cindy. She has been a great help to me in writing this book. It amazes me that there are so many smart, alert, hard-working, dedicated, younger people who are making the world a smarter, better, and more knowledgeable place to live.

About the Cover

Dr. Joanna Budwig made some of the greatest cancer discoveries of all time. She was a biochemist who found some severe discrepancies in the red blood cells of cancer patients. She devised a technique to analyze a cancer patient's blood fat metabolism. What she found was a revelation in cancer research. Using her microscope, Dr. Budwig found that the blood in cancer patients had a greenish color. She then found that the color came from blood platelet coagulation (sticky blood), pictured on the cover. Her analysis then led her to discover that almost every cancer patient had coagulated (sticky) blood. This was keeping the red blood cells from carrying oxygen to the body cells. From those findings, she made some revolutionary discoveries. All of this information can be found in chapter 1 of the book.

Another two very important paradigms in curing cancer are the Cell-Sonic Very Intense Pressure Pulse therapy machine, and the Onnetsu 4 in 1 therapy machine (center photo on cover). The Budwig clinic in Spain uses both therapy machines to help cure cancer. Along with the other procedures being used, the Budwig clinic has a very high cure rate for cancer. They plan to open a new clinic in Florida.

These machines also cure many other diseases including kidney stones, wound healing, enlarged prostate, gall stones, rheumatic arthritis, prostate cancer, breast cancer, and many other diseases. These treatment options are very promising. Don't miss these three chapters, chapters 1, 12, and 38.

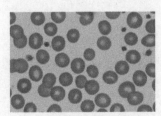

Free Blood

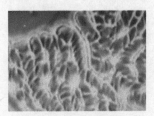

Sticky Blood

Foreword

Helping People Prevent and Cure Cancer

My mission in life is to help people who want to prevent cancer and/or help those to cure cancer. For more than 35 years I have given hundreds of courses on orthodontics, temporal mandibular joint treatment, nutrition, cancer treatment, and cognitive thinking.

Being a cancer advisor, I realize that every person is the author of their destiny. The decisions on what you eat and drink plus your lifestyle determines the health of your blood, cells, organs, and brain. What I see more than anything else is that preventing cancer is a lifetime daily effort, not just for today. Most cancers are predestined to start many years from the date when they are found. Most cancers begin and progress from a chronic lifetime diet of poor eating and lifestyle habits.

What people need to realize is that diet diligence should be practiced every day. I didn't realize that until I was over 35 years old. Younger people think that they will live forever and that a little non-compliance will not hurt anyone. But when you get older, you will realize, that is not always the case.

Most cancers begin from many years of chronic consumption of sugars, sugar products, red meats, preservatives, vegetable oils on the grocery shelf, processed and refined foods. Cancer is not usually found until the cancer cells have been in the body for over 36 months. It is a matter of life and death once it has been diagnosed. No matter what age you are, the time to start preventing cancer is today. If you are younger, please begin to acquire good eating and drinking habits. It will be the greatest thing you could ever do for your health and longevity. When a person gets older, most of them say, "I wish I had kept better care of myself." Why did I buy all those refined and processed foods, etc.?

If you have any questions about preventing or treating cancer, please visit my newsletter website at preventingcancer.substack.com/about. I will be glad to answer any questions to the best of my knowledge. If you have any friends, relatives, or neighbors who would like to get this book, please give them my email or phone address. I also produce a weekly preventive cancer BULLETIN. If you would like to receive it each week, please contact me. My wish for you is to lead a very learning, healthful, happy, exciting, and wonderful life.

About the Author

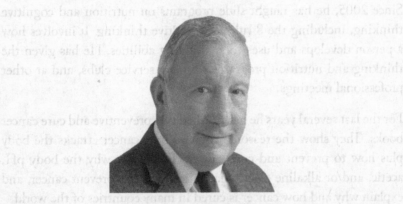

Dr. Loudon graduated from Central Washington University in 1954. In 1957 he graduated from the University of Washington School of Dentistry. He spent two years in the air force as an air force dentist at the San Antonio air defense command, until 1959

In 1959, he moved back to the Wenatchee, Washington area, and set up a dental office in East Wenatchee. He practiced on the same street in East Wenatchee for 45 years.

His office treated patients for general dentistry, orthodontics, and temporal mandibular joint dysfunction (TMD) treatment.

In 1970, he started teaching twelve, and 18-day courses in orthodontics, TMD treatment, and nutrition. He has lectured extensively in Canada, the United States, England, Australia, South Korea, Hong Kong, and many other countries. In 1982 he invented a procedure that corrects and eliminates otitis media, an infection of the inner ear (eustachian tube) in children. His procedure included putting composite tops on the deciduous 1st and 2nd mandibular primary molars, which also corrects and prevents many over closed children and future temporal mandibular dysfunction patients. The procedure also eliminates the need to put in eardrum tubes (grommets), saving 3 % to 5 % of hearing loss when tubes are placed. Otitis media relief is usually obtained in 24 to 48 hours.

In 2014, he taught a 6 day, orthodontic, TMD dysfunction treatment, and nutrition course in Cairo, Egypt.

Since 2005, he has taught slide programs on nutrition and cognitive thinking, including the 8 rules of cognitive thinking. It involves how a person develops and uses their thinking abilities. He has given the thinking and nutrition programs to many service clubs, and at other professional meetings.

For the last several years he has finished two preventive and cure cancer books. They show the reasons why and how cancer attacks the body plus how to prevent and cure cancer. They show why the body pH, acetic, and/or alkaline electromagnetic foods can prevent cancer, and explain why and how cancer is cured in many countries of the world.

The books offer alternative new and proven ways that alternative cancer clinics, cancer physicians, and cancer therapists prevent and cure cancer.

Check out and Subscribe to my Newsletter:

Visit us

Preface

There are a great many ways to treat cancer and other major diseases. My older brother has had non-Hodgkins lymphoma for the last five years. He has been having an IV blood transfusion once a week for about four hours. The cost of this treatment is about $14,000.00 per month. Over the last five years, his medical bills have been over $500,000.00. Many cancer victims decide that they cannot afford the cost of cancer treatment, especially if their medical insurance does not pay the major cost.

But all is not lost. In this book, there are over 22+ major alternate functional medicine cancer treatments where cancer patients have had great success in curing cancer. These treatments come from all over the world. The treatments will reduce and help cure cancer, at a far less gamble and cost. There is one cancer rule, however, ALL of the treatments need to be used as a unit. The first five treatments in chapter 8 are CRITICAL PROCEDURES that should be urgent, even if you are using the oncologists for curing your cancer.

If a cancer patient skips any of the 22+ procedures, the chances of curing cancer will rapidly diminish. Some of the procedures can be fairly expensive, but not nearly as expensive as chemo, radiation, and or surgery. Your future life is the ultimate goal.

If the cancer patient desires, these cancer treatments also can be used with chemotherapy, radiation, chemo drugs, and sometimes surgery. With chemo, far less dosage needs to be used. My suggestion is to pick a friend to help you.

Many new cancer treatments have been introduced in the last few years that will lessen the gamble for alternative cancer patient's survival and in saving lives. The future holds a lot of promise, and a cancer patient today should learn about the treatments needed to save lives or go where cancer clinics are saving lives, like the Budwig cancer clinic in Spain. This book may help you save your own life.

Contents

Introduction

For the last 70 years, cancer treatment in the United States has had almost no change. Four methods that have been used, chemotherapy, radiation, chemotherapy drugs, and surgery. In these many years, the treatments have not changed very much.

There has been an alternative metabolic method to cure cancer in the U.S., but it has been subdued and pushed aside by the medical establishment. With the present medical establishment's cancer modalities, the success rate for curing cancer for over 5 years is about 55 percent. It may be higher with some cancers.

In the U.S., and all over the world, alternative cancer physicians have been using more homeopathic alternate ways to cure cancer. Their cancer cure rate is close to 85 to 90 percent. Yet, in the United States, the average success rate by the medical establishment is close to 55 percent. With some cancers, it is now a little higher. The cancer treatment costs for all cancer patients in the U.S. is estimated at 200 billion dollars per year.

With the present cancer treatments by the medical establishment, the success rates for cancer may not change very much in the future, because they do not let many other cancer treatments to be used, except their patented drugs.

In this book, I have listed more than TWENTY-TWO cancer treatments, used all over the world to cure cancer, even grade III and IV cancers. They need to be used as an intensive COMPLETE THERAPY. Be sure to read about all of them in the following chapters and Chapter 39.

There are many basic cancer cure treatments in this book, used all over the world, with great success. These many homeopathic alternate treatment systems are used to cure cancer. They need to be used as a total unit. if a cancer patient does not follow the rules, the cancer patient is playing Russian roulette with their life.

Many very successful treatments are in this book. The treatments in this book are noninvasive, and also can be used with chemotherapy, radiation, chemotherapy drugs, and surgery. Most oncologists will not mention any other treatments, even though they are direly needed.

A few oncologists are now lowering their dosage of chemo drugs and using many of these alternate cancer therapies. Recently, reports have come out that vitamin C, I. V. is one of those treatments, along with I. V. laetrile. Most oncologists do not use any other treatments except the four basic therapies.

Joanna Budwig's cottage cheese, flaxseed oil, quark, crushed flaxseed formula, PANCREATIC ENZYMES, the CellSonic electro-hydraulic therapy machine, and four in one therapy, are examples of treatments that should be given to every cancer patient. There are many more listed that would HELP cure cancer. They are highlighted in chapters 8, 9, 10, 12, and 39.

Every cancer patient, even if using the oncologist's treatment, should be made aware of, and use these alternate cancer treatments. They could still have the oncologist's usual chemotherapy, radiation, chemotherapy drugs, and surgery if they prefer.

It may be very wise to look into many of these therapies, including many mentioned in this book. Cancer treatment clinics like Dr. Joanna Budwig's clinic in Spain, plus others, in the U.S., Canada, and Mexico claim a very high success rate for curing cancer. For those that choose an alternate treatment, they must seriously follow every rule that is laid out, and not miss any of the mentioned treatments. Any negligence may end in failure and possible loss of life. All available knowledge about cancer treatment should be gained by the cancer victim, so they will be able to make the right intelligent decisions.

Cancer tests will also be a way to find out if a person has cancer before it is detected by the medical establishment. Better cancer tests are coming online, and are available. From the time a cancer cell is started in the body, it is about 36 months before most of them are detected by the oncologist. That is why it is so important to find a cancer tumor before it is diagnosed. Tests will soon be able to do that.

My Sad Story about Prostate Cancer Treatment

When I started this book, I wanted to prevent prostate cancer victims, from undergoing the sad experience that I went through with prostate cancer. My prostate cancer was detected just AFTER proton therapy was being introduced. At the time I also did not know the wonderful non-invasive formulas, supplements, procedures, and treatments in this book.

My older brother had surgery to remove his prostate when they found his PSI was greatly elevated. He suggested that I have prostate surgery for my prostate condition. That was one of the biggest mistakes of my life. My physician did not explain the problems that would exist after I had prostate surgery. There was nothing said about not being able to have an erection, incontinence, and having to wear pads for the rest of my life. At the time, proton radiation therapy was being used in Loma Linda, and If I would have known, that would have been my choice. No physician mentioned proton therapy, or diet instructions, what to eat, what not to eat, or anything else.

Many prostate options can prevent prostate removal. I would not advise any man to create the problems that I am going through. The present problems of incontinence will be with me forever.

I would not recommend prostate removal surgery as an option for prostate cancer treatment unless it was the only option. I think that there are many options and great cancer treatments that can now be used.

Foreword

by Professor Andrew Hague,
Acta Scientific Cancer Biology

You bought this book because you or your loved ones are scared you may be killed by cancer. This is not a book for entertainment or extending your knowledge; it is a lifesaver. Dr. Loudon has put his heart into it, so to speak, based on his suffering and considerable medical experience. Follow the advice here, and you will be safer than any other method offered to you.

Hopefully, you are wanting to prevent cancer and have not yet been diagnosed. Cancer can be prevented, and diet is essential. We are what we eat. This book is aimed mostly at rich countries, where the food quality is generally low due to overprocessing. It is a calamity that countries that think they are the most civilized have worse food typically eaten by hunter-gatherers in the jungle. There could almost be a rule that if advertised and packed in a colorful carton, don't trust it.

Dr. Loudon's advice is essential for everyone. Even for those not worried about cancer, healthy living is essential. I have long since thought about writing a book on "Survival in a Civilised Society." The dangers in modern life are huge, from earning money to keeping it, traveling safely, meeting strangers, knowing who to trust, and then knowing how to keep our bodies healthy. The chapter on health is already written thanks to Dr. Loudon, and it is in this book that you have wisely selected.

As you proceed, chapter by chapter, you will wonder how ignorance of cancer prevention has come about. Soon you will realize that cancer is the biggest scam in history. Ask yourself, who likes cancer? It is Big Pharma, the manufacturers of chemotherapy drugs banned in warfare and legal in hospitals. Chemotherapy and mustard gas are the same. It is deadly poisonous. If it can be aimed at cancer cells, it kills them. Often, it also kills healthy cells and usually misses single migrating cancer cells that multiply and grow into large tumors.

What pharmaceutical companies fail to understand is that cancer is not a biochemical problem. Cancer is an electrical fault. It is a biophysical problem. We need physics rather than chemistry to sort out the voltage across the cell. Wounds and cancers are wet cell batteries. Regulating their voltages happens automatically under our immune systems when the immune system is healthy. How to maintain that good governance is what this book tells you.

Recent increases in radio waves for mobile phones and the internet of things have made electrical interference into a medical plague. Studies at Bradford University in England showed that the maximum time for a safe call with a smartphone is six minutes. Beyond that, the brain is damaged incrementally. Each call damages a bit, and those bits add up. If it were an infection, the germs would be found in the blood, and the cause would be apparent. Electrosensitivity is a modern disease, preventable and ignored by politicians, governments, and smartphone addicts. Even town dwellers now enjoying 5G internet connections face damaging electrical waves on every street corner that harm the immune system and prevent it from protecting us against cancer.

There is, unfortunately, an inevitability about cancer. Our body cells replace themselves on average every six weeks. Each new cell should be an exact copy of the cell it replaces. Generally, this works well, but with the billions of replications taking place, a few new cells are different; statistically, mistakes happen. They are mutations, and these are malignant. They replicate profusely, and this is cancer. In a healthy person, the immune system detects the malignant cells. It kills them automatically every day and every night so that those incipient cancers never multiply, and we are unaware of what has happened. We are new, only about 80,000 years old since a brain mutation led to homo sapiens evolving and being different from other similar creatures. Older creatures such as sharks and ants, which have been alive for hundreds of millions of years, do not have cell replication and do not get cancer; their organs are stable.

The next stage of cancer management is to detect incipient tumors by measuring their permittivity. Every person can then be checked twice a year, and cancer stopped before they are aware of it. Dr. Loudon's

22

advice will still be necessary. Do not hope that with a quick cure for cancer, you can gorge on junk. There are plenty of other diseases eager to invade a weakened body. Look at the consequences of obesity and diabetes.

If this book is to be extended, I would add a chapter on exercise. The energy in and energy out is the basis on which we lived as hunter-gatherers for thousands of years until science disrupted our existence, and the word improvement came into our vocabulary. Our bodies have not yet adjusted to modern agriculture and factory processed food. We would need a few more thousand years and many deaths. To enjoy life now, follow Dr. Loudon's advice and become normal like our cave-dwelling ancestors were. This book is not telling you anything new. It is taking you back to before science screwed things up, and now we have to use science to straighten it out safely.

—*Professor Andrew Hague, Acta Scientific Cancer Biology*

1

Dr. Joanna Budwig and
her Incredible Cancer Discoveries

The Greatest Cancer Discovery of all Time

There is one health (cancer) discovery that has a profound health benefit for every living being. This little-known incredible discovery needs to be known and practiced by every person who wants to prevent cancer. It will create great health, less disease, a healthy immune system, and energy-filled life. This discovery has been virtually dormant and unknown since the 1950s when it was discovered.

It begins with Dr. Linus Pauling, a Nobel prize-winning scientist, who has written over 300 scientific books and articles in many scientific fields including quantum chemistry, molecular biology, molecular medicine, physics, and biochemistry. In 1937, Dr. Pauling wrote a book entitled, "The Nature of the Chemical Bonds, and the Structure of Molecules and Crystals." It is still used in college, and medical facilities today. In 1948, Dr. Pauling, with only a piece of paper and a note pad, made a remarkable discovery. He discovered a polypeptide chain formed from amino acids, which would coil into a helix structure called the "alpha helix." It was a globular and fibrous protein that contributed to many advancements in cancer treatment, nutrition, and healing.

Following Dr. Linus Pauling's discoveries, Dr. JoAnna Budwig, a German biochemist, researcher, and pharmacist continued the double helix bond research and made another historic discovery. She found that two essential omega 3 fatty acids, mixed with cottage cheese, formed the double helix bond, and had anti-disease properties, plus a role in curing cancer, preventing sickness, and helping to cure heart disease, strokes, and heart attacks.

She found that linolenic acid (flaxseed oil), mixed with cottage cheese and quark, allows the solution to be water-soluble, can enter into the blood, and body cells to help deliver oxygen, and create electrical energy (pH). She found that the combination not only helped cure most forms of cancer, but is a remarkable cancer cure, and deterrent in preventing many other diseases.

Dr. Budwig's blood discoveries began with her microscope evaluation of the blood in cancer patients. She was the first person to devise a chemical measurement to test blood fat metabolism. She devised a technique to analyze a cancer patient's blood. What she found was a revelation in cancer research. Her new technology soon became a routine that was used around the world.

Dr. Budwig found that the blood in a cancer patient had a strange greenish color. She found that the color came from platelet coagulation (homocysteine laced sticky blood). Her analysis then led her to find that almost every cancer patient's blood was carrying very little oxygen. The coagulation or sticky homocysteine blood was keeping the red blood cells stuck together and not carrying oxygen. The result was that the body and organ cells were being starved of oxygen. This situation was weakening the body cells and the immune system. In turn, the cancer cells love no oxygen, since they multiply and metastasize with a process of glucose metabolism or "glycation." or "glycosylation."

From her biochemistry and physicist knowledge, and examining further, Budwig found that the cause of the oxygen starvation in a cancer patient's blood, came from an excess of omega 6 fatty acids (vegetable oils on the grocery shelf), and sugar. These fatty acids form "transfats" and "mega trans." They come from partially hydrogenated oils in a cancer patient's diet. Since these oils have no electrical charge, they are dead oils and cause a reaction with cancer cell toxins in the blood which restricts the oxygen.

The transfats, mega trans, and sugar were part of the diet a cancer patient eats, which changes the composition of the blood, restricting the electromagnetism, which is absent in the oils. These non-electromagnetic oils on the grocery shelf are also the culprits that cause coagulation in other diseases. They are connected with high blood pressure, heart disease, strokes, heart attacks, and blood clots in the veins, common in diabetes.

Dr. Budwig's incredible discoveries established several very critical and important cancer facts:

1. Almost all cancer patients have blood with a greenish color which comes from sticky red blood cells that were carrying no oxygen.

2. The body cell oxygen starvation paves the way for cancer cells to multiply and metastasize since they need no oxygen. They use sugar, sugar products, carbohydrates, and protein to multiply.

3. Cancer cells love little or no oxygen.

4. The first line of defense for treating cancer should be to unravel coagulated (sticky) blood and take pancreatic enzymes.

5. The first thing any oncologist should do is to inform every cancer patient right away about these important treatments. They seldom do.

6. If you, your neighbor, relative, or friend has cancer, it would be wise to inform them of Dr. Budwig's oxygen starvation of body cells and the unraveling of the sticky blood.

Dr. Budwig's second evolutionary discovery was a food mixture she found that would unravel the greenish coagulated (sticky) blood. Her mixture would unravel the red blood cells, freeing them to carry oxygen to the body cells and the immune system. The formula strengthened the body cells and the immune system, which is direly needed to cure cancer.

Dr. Budwig found that when she mixed cottage cheese, or Quark, cold raw flaxseed oil and crushed raw flaxseeds, it allowed the solution to become water-soluble. Quark is not like plain kefir, because it can produce a reaction of the sulphydryl groups, allowing the flaxseeds to become water-soluble. Kefir and yogurt will not replace Quark or cottage cheese. If you cannot find it, you can make your own. The recipe is easily found on the internet.

Dr. Budwig was so sure that her formula would work on cancer patients that she immediately started treating grade III and grade IV cancer patients at the local hospital. They had been treated previously with chemo and radiation. The oncologists had given up on them and said they had just a few months to live. 2,500 patients later, to their surprise, and with several other cancer modalities, Dr. Budwig got rid of their cancer. 85 to 90 percent of the patients were able to go home and lived for more than 5 years, most of them fully cured.

This is Dr. Budwig's cottage cheese, flaxseed, Quark formula:

1. Start with 2 tablespoons of low-fat milk, 3 tablespoons linseed (flaxseed) oil, which you will mix with a Wisk type mixer or electric stick type blender until it is nice and smooth. (An electric blender is preferred as you can be sure the oil blends well with all the other ingredients.).

2. Next, add 1 teaspoon of honey and mix all 3 ingredients.

3. Now slowly add the low-fat Quark or cottage cheese, 2 tablespoons at a time, and keep mixing until it is mixed well, putting in a total of 6 level tablespoons of low-fat Quark/cottage cheese (must be 2% fat or less.)

4. In a separate bowl put 2 tablespoons of freshly crushed flaxseeds that you have ground up with a coffee grinder.

5. Now put some fruit (berries, lemons, nuts, etc, over the flaxseeds).

6. Then finally pour the mixture of Quark, honey, and oil over the flaxseeds and fruit. That is the original way that Dr. Budwig liked to prepare it for her patients. Cancer patients received this formula every day.

This is a great preventive cancer formula for those that want to prevent cancer and heart disease. It can be taken every morning if desired.

For prevention, and If you have cancer, there are at least six other critical and essential rules you need to follow with Dr. Budwig's formula to stay disease and cancer-free. See my list of 22 cancer treatment remedies in chapters 8, 9, and 10.

1. Reduce or stop eating all sugar, candy, and sugar products.

2. Reduce or stop all DEEP FRIED and fried foods, where (cooked) oils from the grocery shelf are used.

3. Reduce or stop all red meats.

4. Reduce or stop all refined, and processed foods.

5. Get 15 to 30 minutes of sunshine if possible, 10,000 iu of Vit. D3, 2,000 mg of vitamin C, natural acerola (not ascorbic acid), zinc, and exercise every day.

6. With cancer, get some solozymes from www.collegehealth-stores.com and take 12 to 18 each day between meals. This is very critical.

7. Eat two to four crushed cloves of black fermented garlic every day. (this type leaves no odor and is more effective than regular garlic.

8. Eat 8 to 12 or more raw, fresh vegetables, fruits, berries, melons, bulb and / or leaves.

There you have it. I know of an alternative cancer doctor who has been taking Joanna Budwig's formula every morning for 12 years. He has had no colds, sickness, or health problems for all of those years. My wife and I have been taking her formula for over two years. We are planning to take it every day for the rest of our lives.

I feel this is "The Greatest Cancer Discovery of all Time."

2

Pancreatic Enzymes:
Why you Need Them to Cure Cancer

When I talk about pancreatic enzymes, I have to start with an orthodontist that I met in Texas, many years ago. His name was Dr. William
Kelley. Dr. Kelley had a wonderful wife, four beautiful children, and
a great thriving orthodontic practice. He had medical training in the
Navy before going to college and dental school.

While in dental school, he also worked in the electro cardiac department at the local hospital. During that time, he also took a nutrition
course in dental school, read many nutrition books, and understood a
great amount of nutrition knowledge.

Four years after beginning his orthodontic practice in Texas, he began
to lose energy, and just felt bad. Over the next two years, he felt worse
and worse, until he had to rest between patients for him to proceed.
It was then that he found he had metastasized terminal cancer in his
pancreas and liver. His cancer was so advanced that they thought if
they did the surgery, he might die on the operating table. They gave
him only two to four months to live.

With his medical training and his research into enzymes, by Dr. John
Beard, he started taking massive amounts of pancreatic enzymes. He
found that he had to detoxify himself with coffee enemas while changing his diet. He then started taking a large number of enzymes, vitamins, amino acids, and minerals.

Dr. Kelley started feeling better and better. Because of his knowledge,
research, diet, and enzymes, he cured himself of one of the worst forms
of cancer.

After getting back to his office full time, cancer and other disease patients asked him to help them. Soon, he had cured more and more cancer patients, as well as those with diabetes, heart disease, and other ailments. After a time, he had cured thousands of cancer and other disease patients.

Another exciting chapter in Dr. Kelley's life occurred when a very bright medical student, Dr. Nicholas Gonzalez read about Dr. Kelley and his success with curing cancer. With approval from his superior, Dr. Gonzalez proceeded to investigate this "fraud" as far as the medical profession was concerned. Dr. Gonzalez went to Texas and began to examine Dr. Kelley's records on these cancer patients. To his surprise, they were extremely accurate and truthful. Dr. Kelley kept immaculate records on the many thousands of cancer patients he had cured. Dr. Gonzalez wrote up the records on 50+ of Dr. Kelley's cured patients, later writing a book about Dr. Kelley's success.

This changed the way that Dr. Gonzalez thought about curing cancer. The proof was enough that when Dr. Gonzalez graduated from medical school, he started using Dr. Kelley's program in treating cancer with this great alternative cancer treatment. During the next decade, Dr. Gonzalez cured about 85 to 90 percent of his cancer patients (over 10,000) using Dr. Kelley's program, plus using some of his additional treatments. Unfortunately, Dr. Gonzalez died in 2018, along with about 77 other alternative cancer doctors who also mysteriously died between 2015 and 2019. Dr. Gonzalez's book, "One Man alone," is a great story of Dr. Kelley and one that every professional should get and read. It can be found on Amazon.com.

Dr. Kelley's story is also written in a book called "Victory over Cancer." It was written by Dr. Kelley and Fred Rahe. The book begins with his life story, his treatment, and how he cured his cancer. It is a revelation of how cancer can be cured. It is also a great story about why pancreatic enzymes are one of the great treatments used to cure cancer. This should be a "must-read" for serious professionals. and cancer victims. It can be obtained by calling 623 327 1778, or from his website at www. drkelley.info.

I will list a few of the important issues related to enzymes and the treatment of cancer. Cancer is an ectopic germ cell mutating into the wrong place. It is common in pregnant women when they first get conceived, but cures itself with pancreatic enzymes in the uterus.

Cancer usually starts in an acidic body with an insufficient amount of enzymes to digest excess amounts of protein. It usually starts with a "hit" in the body cell mitochondria from an overworked pancreas due to excessive amounts of protein, sugar, vegetable oils, and other acidic foods. The pancreas can only produce small amounts of enzymes, not enough for excess eating of those foods.

Dr. Kelley made a great comparison of diabetes and cancer. He stated: "Diabetes is a disorder of sugar and carbohydrate metabolism due to inadequate production and/or utilization of insulin. Cancer is a disorder of protein metabolism due to inadequate production and/or utilization of protein, and digestive enzymes." These enzymes Kelley mentioned are produced by the pancreas.

Dr. Kelley stated that massive amounts of these pancreatic enzymes produce very good results. The enzymes that he is referring to are pig enzymes and are very hard to get. They are called solozymes. These same enzymes are used now by many European and alternative U.S. cancer physicians, plus many alternative metabolic cancer doctors in the U.S. These pancreatic enzymes can be obtained from www.college-healthstores.com or by calling 817 458 9241.

The action of enzymes: Enzymes are produced by the pancreas to help digest the food that enters the small intestine. These enzymes can be absorbed through the wall of the small intestine, travel in the blood. and go to the cancer cells. One of these enzymes is trypsin, which can travel in the blood to the tumor. How does it destroy cancer cells? It can tell the difference between good cells and cancer cells because of the low electrical properties and valence of the cancer cells. At the CANCER SITE, and IN THE BLOOD, it breaks down the tumor cells. Trypsin cannot break down the cancer cells by itself. It needs other pancreatic enzymes to help kill the cancer cells. Many years ago, Dr. John Beard used enzyme injections directed into the cancer cells, which digested the cancer tumor. But Dr. Kelley found that oral enzymes work just as well, with less trauma.

Another less potent enzyme formula can be very effective in preventing cancer and can be found on Amazon.com. It is called wobenzym-N. Wobenzym-N is made in Florida, and has many pancreatic enzymes, but does not work as good as solozymes. It also can be a substitute for solozymes if they are not available. For cancer, a patient would need 15 to 18 each day between meals, the same as solozymes. For prevention, three to five Wobenzym-N tablets a day would be just the right amount.

Cancer cells make their enzymes. The enzyme that cancer cells make is called "malignin." The malignin digests body cell protein around the cancer cells. The more malignin that the cancer cells can produce, the faster the cancer cells grow. Enzymes are part of a four-prong master list in curing cancer. There are many other things that I have mentioned in the four-part "Cause, Prevention, and cure for cancer." These most important four things are, Dr. Joanna Budwig's cottage cheese, flaxseed oil formula, pancreatic enzymes, the CellSonic electrohydraulic therapy machine, and the 4 in 1 therapy machine, used by the Budwig cancer clinic in Spain now, but hopefully will be approved by the FDA for use in the U.S. The FDA needs to give the OK for using the CellSonic machine for cancer, plus the 4 in 1 Therapy machine. I think they will eventually get approval in the U.S. A person with cancer, cannot forget to use the many other critical treatments that I mention in chapters 8, 9, 10, and 39 of the book.

3

Basic Principles in the Cause of Cancer

Cancer is a terrible disease. To understand how to prevent cancer or cure it, a person can better understand the disease by learning what the basic elements are that cause cancer. These are the atoms and atom groups involved with the molecules that make up the food we eat and the cells of the human body. The atoms in food and the body are in two forms, anionic atoms and cationic atoms, called anions and cations. An anion is an atom that is negatively charged and has more electrons than protons in the nucleus. The electrons rotate clockwise. A cation is an atom (or groups of atoms) that is positively charged and the electrons rotate in a counter-clockwise rotation.

Why am I starting here? Because the following information is the basic formula for energy. What is energy? It is the strength and vitality required for physical and mental metabolism or metabolism of and in the human body. All living forms need electromagnetism, energy, vitality, and strength to live and survive. The anionic and cationic actions, when associated together, will give a person the capacity to stay healthy, and/or in the wrong circumstances, become unhealthy. Are you still with me? Putting this scenario in perspective is very important. All foods are composed of ELECTROMAGNETIC ANIONS, or NON, ELECTRO-MAGNETIC CATIONS. These two types of foods, anions, and cations, WHEN COMBINED, produce the energy for our bodies. The human body needs way more anionic foods than unhealthy cationic foods to stay healthy.

Where are anionic foods? They are found in plants raised in the soil, where they can get the minerals, amino acids, vitamins, and nutrients needed for humans to stay healthy. However, they are not anionic until they are eaten and get into the digestive tract. Once eaten, the EN-ZYMES that digest them are anionic. When they are mixed (live raw

34

plant food, enzymes, and vitamins), the foods become anionic. On the other side, cationic foods are foods that have no energy. They are ALTERED FOODS (refined, processed) from the anionic plants, trees, minerals, and other anionic sources. What are the cationic non- electromagnetic foods? They are refined and processed foods, sugar, all oils on the grocery shelf except extra virgin olive oil, red meat oils, preservatives, GMO foods, overcooked anionic foods, etc. These cationic foods also produce an acidic environment.

Now, for another explanation. Dr. Carey Reams, a chemist who worked with biological ionization of the body, found that all foods except the lemon were cationic (the minerals, calcium, and potassium are also anionic). Most cationic foods cannot become anionic, because they have no electromagnetic energy. Like I mentioned, in the digestive tract, when alkaline anionic enzymes are added, the live foods become anionic. But what if the non, electromagnetic, cationic foods outnumber the electromagnetic anionic foods? That is where the TROUBLE STARTS. The cationic foods produce little or NO ENERGY.

An overload of these cationic culprits (refined, processed, and altered foods), create havoc in the lower intestine. You have 25+ trillion little creatures there that need to be fed live anionic food. That keeps the ratio of good bacteria to bad bacteria in the small intestine at a healthy ratio or about 80 good to 20 percent bad bacteria. When the cationic foods (which produce no energy), increase to a nasty (more than 20 percent) ratio, bad bacteria, maybe a 70 to 30 percent ratio, or worse, there is trouble in River City. These nasty bad bacteria overwhelm the good bacteria and create toxins and inflammation that break down the small intestinal wall (called leaky gut) and sneak through into the blood. That is the origin of autoimmune and other diseases.

Another equation needs to be entered here. Most ANIONIC electromagnetic foods are alkaline. Most CATIONIC non, electromagnetic foods are acidic. These anionic foods in the intestines are alkaline after the enzymes are mixed. This acid, base balance ratio also needs to be at an optimal amount and balanced for maintaining a healthy body. The ratio can vary from very acidic to very alkaline. The anionic/cationic, acid/base balance then, or pH, can be measured with hydrion litmus paper. It can be obtained at health food stores, or on the internet. The optimum body, cell acid/base range is measured by hydrion litmus paper. Optimum urine and saliva should be 6.2 to 6.8 pH (optimum health, 6.4 pH). This is the ideal energy range for optimum health, vitality, and a disease-free state.

Anionic body (neutral pH) molecules and anionic (neutral pH) bacteria (80+ percent) in the small intestine provide us with energy, vitality, strength, free from diseases, and most cancers. To summarize, live RAW vegetables, fruits, grains, legumes, nuts, berries, leaves, bulbs, and minerals are the anionic foundation for good health. When the CATIONIC, acetic, non, electromagnetic, acetic food ratio goes to the cationic side, many diseases begin to creep into the body. This includes cancer. The toxins in the small intestine disrupt the bacteria ratio and produce toxins and inflammation of the small intestinal wall. This leads to *leaky gut (open holes)* that go into the blood. Bad bacteria, protein particles, toxins, and parasite larvae then get in the blood. They can even go to the brain. With an acetic CATIONIC, low body cell pH, bad culprits can spread into the blood, and the body cells, changing the cell RNA, and the DNA in the mitochondria. This causes a mitochondria "hit," and the beginning of cancer.

36

4

The Most Important and Unique Wall in the World

The most important and unique wall in the world is the one to two-celled thin intestinal lining of your small intestine (gut wall). It is responsible for keeping you healthy and determines the health of your body cells, organs, blood, heart, and even your brain. It not only determines the health and protects your body, but your ability to resist disease, also to think, adjust your heartbeat, and most of all your ability to live a long and prosperous life.

A reservoir of dendritic cells patrols the border of your gut wall. Chemicals called cytokines are released when toxins cause inflammation. They send macrophages to combat the toxins and protect the intestinal cell wall. What makes the intestinal wall so important is that the cytokines, macrophages, and healthy bacteria (healthy microbiome) control the gut lining to keep it healthy. With a healthy gut wall, the healthy bacteria transfer minerals, vitamins, enzymes, amino acids, and other nutrients, through the thin cell gut walls and into the blood. In the blood, these nutrients do their magic and go to all the body cells and organs, keeping the body healthy and free of disease (with a good diet). It all relates to the healthy gut microbes being vital and healthy from a great diet and lifestyle. These 25+ trillion good, healthy bacteria are a person's greatest bosom friends.

When the diet is not good, and a person has a chronic consumption of sugars, omega 6 vegetable oils, red meat, refined, and processed foods, etc., things do not go so well. There is trouble in River City. The colonies of inflammatory toxins from the bad diet, create inflammation, and holes in the very thin gut wall. They overwhelm the cytokines and macrophages. The dam breaks, opening the intestinal wall gate to bad terrorists (tiny food molecules, proteins, bad bacteria, molds, parasite larvae, candida fungus, and disease. These holes even can get bigger as the inflammatory toxins continue to erode the thin walls, and deregulate the gut. This next part is scary. The endotoxins, bad bacteria, fungus, parasite larvae, and polysaccharides that escape into your blood can travel to your heart, body cells, organs, and brain. This is the start of chronic disease, including autoimmune diseases plus serious ailments like HBP, heart disease, diabetes, cancer, and brain disorders.

Microglial cells protect your brain from infections. The brain has a blood-brain barrier like the small intestinal lining. The lymph system takes out the waste. But here is the bad part. Microglial cells are the primary immune cells of the central nervous system. They act like cytokines and macrophages, responding to toxic pathogens, and injury. An invasion of toxic chemical toxins can overpower the microglial cells. The microglial brain cells get overwhelmed. Certain toxic bacteria and toxic molecules then breach the blood-brain barrier and enter the brain.

Recent research has shown that although microglial and t-cells try to suppress inflammation in the brain, a swarm of inflammation toxins can pass through the blood-brain barrier and overwhelm the neurons, axons, and synapses. The synapse creates chemical reactions involving acetylcholine to communicate and function between nerve cells. Chemical damage to the synapse occurs and is critical in altering brain function. It is now found that depression, dementia, Alzheimer's disease, Parkinson's disease, multiple sclerosis, sleep deprivation, and some other brain functions are all related to this debilitating toxic chemical disease process. It all starts with a leaky gut in the small intestine, when the toxins, bad bacteria, and other nasty culprits travel in the blood to the brain.

It all starts with the intestinal wall lining. That is why it is so important to have a good diet. It can be said that 90 percent of all diseases start with a bad diet. The inflammatory toxins that breach the gut lining create havoc on the joints, body cells, organs, heart, and even the brain. A healthy diet keeps the thin small intestinal walls strong and toxin resistant. That is why the gut wall is the most important and unique in the world. It also proves that the health of the small intestinal wall determines the health of the body cells, white blood cells, and the brain. If more people knew this, there would be more healthy brains, and a lot less depression, dementia, Alzheimer's disease, Parkinson's disease, multiple sclerosis, sleep deprivation, and other brain function issues.

5

Ninety Percent of all Diseases
Start in The Small Intestine

The good healthy bacteria in your small intestine control your health, immunity, disease control, energy, brain health, and even your longevity. Mark Hyman, M.D. is an expert on intestinal bacteria, and he says, "the bacteria, viruses, and fungi which make up your intestinal flora (microbiome) control your life, immune system, disease, and cancer prevention. The answer to a disease-free, life is not to eliminate bacteria, but to instead make food choices that promote a healthy colony of gut bacteria."

But it is getting harder and harder to get good healthy bacteria in the foods that we eat. Good healthy bacteria are nurtured from the soil. The soil is being used more and more, losing nutrients in the food that make up your health. More and more pesticides, roundup, and GMO sprays are also competing with the health of your gut bacteria. The 67 minerals that make up your gut bacteria and body are being depleted more and more.

What are the healthy choices that Dr. Mark Hyman is talking about? They are in the foods that we buy and eat every day. Now, 94 percent of all corn and soy products have been exposed to GMO chemicals. Corn and soy are also genetically modified. Many other foods have also been exposed to pesticides and GMO substances. With these unfavorable changes in the production of our food, it leaves us with some important decisions on what we buy and eat.

Here are some suggestions on getting and eating the food that is most important for your gut bacteria, immune system, and prevention of cancer.

1. Most important, buy foods that are organic, electromagnetic, raw, and fresh. Most diseases are caused by a bad diet of sugar products, omega 6 vegetable oils, refined, and processed foods.

2. Make your soups from the raw, fresh foods that you buy, or from fresh frozen vegetables and fruits. Commercially canned soups, processed meats, and other canned foods contain many preservatives, fructose, corn syrup, sodium phosphate, potassium chloride, hydrolyzed soy protein, and many other ingredients that are not good for your gut bacteria. I know that they are easy and fast to prepare, but not the best for your health.

3. A great option is to plant your garden or think about it very seriously. For about 30 years I have planted a garden every year. My garden is in two small plots, only about 3 feet by 8 feet. Yet I grow enough carrots, beets, cucumbers, kohlrabi, and tomatoes to eat, from July to the last of October. Next to my house, I grow acorn squash and radishes. Other vegetables, fruits, squash, legumes, berries, plants, and other raw fresh things, I buy (mostly organic) at the grocery store. Another option is to make your soups from leftover salad makings and freeze them. That way you know what is in them, what ingredients are in them, and that they are not filled with preservatives and unwanted foods.

4. In the grocery store, stay away from the tantalizing rows of chips, refined, processed foods, sugar, corn syrup, fructose filled, or coated products, plus vegetable oils on the grocery shelf, especially GMO raised canola oil, corn oil, and margarine. You may make an exception of extra virgin olive oil, as it may be on the grocery shelf but should be in the refrigerator, or it will turn to an omega 6 oil. But remember, flaxseed oil, Udo's choice, fish oils, cod liver oil, and northern seed oils are a much better form of polyunsaturated oils than extra virgin olive oil. Make sure you have these in your refrigerator and get 2 tablespoons a day.

5. Avoid deep-fried oils in restaurants. Most deep-frying oils, used for French fries, fish, and chicken, are vegetable oils that are non-electromagnetic (dead) oils. They help destroy the good bacteria in your small intestine. Restaurants use them because they are cheap and can be used over and over. These deep-frying oils, when consumed, turn into "trans

fats and mega trans," which form homocysteine (sticky) blood, causing clots in your blood, strokes, heart attacks, and cancer.

6. Minimize your consumption of wieners, sausage, bacon, and other processed meats. The preservatives, nitrates, and often, fructose, or sugar coatings are very bad, and evil foods for your gut bacteria. You can eat some at picnics and gatherings unless you have cancer. Try to use them sparingly.

7. Don't skip fermented foods. Gut bacteria love fermented foods. Kimchi, kombucha, sauerkraut, kefir, and cottage cheese, are some of the most welcome foods for your bacterial guests.

8. Most people do not think about tests to check on their intestinal bacteria. However, with artificial intelligence, the tests will help anyone with discomfort and intestinal problems. A spectrum of blood, urine, stool, and even breath tests can detect many digestive problems like leaky gut, ulcerative colitis, Crohn's disease, leukocytosis, and others. With the help of artificial intelligence in the future, these diseases will be easier to detect and cure. Preventive physicians and naturopaths are beginning to give these tests.

By now, you are probably saying. "What can I eat to keep my gut bacteria happy, wise, and healthy?" Here are some other great food reminders that your intestinal guests will be very happy to receive. Raw or lightly cooked fresh broccoli, cabbage, cauliflower, spinach, kohlrabi, onions, garlic (crushed), asparagus, lentils, peas, beans, kale, white cheese, fermented foods, chicken, wild fish (not farmed), omega 3 oils, leeks, white cheese, kefir, rye bread, turmeric, L-arginine, vitamin D3, vitamin C, selenium, raw almonds, pecans, walnuts, pistachios, cucumbers, radishes, beets, squash, berries, cottage cheese, spinach, and all other raw plants, seeds, plus other good supplements.

6

Six Reasons why Toxins, Inflammation, and Leaky Gut will Cause Disease and Cancer

Much of the food we eat today is far different than the foods we ate just thirty years ago. Every year, more chemicals, pesticides, preservatives, and additives are added to our food supply. Many places where food is grown, has been depleted of the minerals needed for good health. It is hard to get the great foods that keep your intestinal bacteria healthy and maintain a great immune system.

One of the reasons cancer has become so rampant is the reduction of nutrients from the soil and the use of pesticides, chemicals, preservatives, sugar, sugar products, carbohydrates, excess red meat, and omega 6 oils in our foods. These products cause diseases and cancer.

There are many food guidelines available in magazines and emails that a person receives every week, but not everyone has the time to read them. I would like to dwell on six of the multiple reasons why toxins, inflammation, and leaky gut cause autoimmune and other diseases including cancer. The list will cover the dirty dozen (foods with the most pesticides and chemicals), fewer pesticides and not so good chemicals, processed foods, GMO foods, animals raised in pens, fish, and fowl, plus cancer-causing foods.

The pluses of raw fresh foods overshadow the negatives when it comes to health.

1. The sprayed foods: These are foods containing the most toxins from pesticides and chemicals. It is wise to buy these foods organic if possible. Cherries, grapes, apples, celery, green, col-

ored peppers, fresh corn, cabbage, pears, nectarines, and peaches. Always wash foods with H2O2 or soda water.

2. Foods with fewer pesticides and chemicals. These have fewer contaminants. If you can, these can also be bought organic. Broccoli, cauliflower, brussels sprouts, asparagus, cantaloupe, watermelon, onions, pineapple, kiwi, bananas, fresh peas, beans, kohlrabi, beets, and radishes. Wash thoroughly with H2O2 or soda water.

3. Processed and refined foods. These foods are not good for the bacteria in your gut. They compromise the immune system and are right in the middle of the disease and the cancer center ring. The processed foods contain nitrates, preservatives, corn syrup, fructose, artificial coloring, stabilizers, flavor additives, and many other chemicals. My advice is that for picnics, and family affairs, they may be permissible, but go easy on other days.

4. GMO foods: By now, almost everyone knows that in the U.S., corn and soy are 90+ percent genetically modified. Also, most grain crops are sprayed with glyphosate (roundup) to dry the crops and kill pests. Corn and soy products are all over the grocery shelves, but the FDA does not have to have any labels that state they are GMO. Corn chips, Fritos, corn breakfast cereals, and Tostitos are all GMO products. Roundup has now been proven to cause cancer in humans. Be careful, if you buy these products.

5. PEN raised fish, animals, and birds: They all contain antibodies, hormones, antibiotics, and other chemicals, from the food that they are eating. The meat of most pen-raised animals contains up to 30 percent more omega 6 fat. Some omega 6 fat will not hurt you, but the amount in animals, if eaten regularly, may. Wild raised fish, animals, and birds, are much better for your health.

6. Disease, and cancer, causing foods. The keys to preventing disease and cancer are to prevent toxins, inflammation of the intestinal wall, and leaky gut, to invade your blood, and body

cells. Some foods also produce toxins, which have a link to autoimmune and other diseases, including cancer. These are GMO sugar beets, made into sugar, sugar products, boiled, and deep-frying vegetable oils on the grocery shelf (except extra virgin olive oil), excess red meat (very acidic), regular soda drinks, diet soda, preservatives, and aspartame.

There are also some important ways to help prevent disease and cancer. Some of these are:

1. To reduce stress. Researchers are finding that stress is one of the factors that is linked to cancer. Depression, stress, and worry are harmful to your health.

2. Find time for relaxation, meditation, read, get a hobby, or just hang out.

3. Take supplements: These are some of the things that help eliminate toxins.

Vitamin C, D3, folic acid, B6, B12, L-arginine, ginkgo Biloba, glutathione, CoQ10, selenium, zinc, turmeric, and ginger.

4. Fermented foods and probiotics; I would heartily recommend kimchi, sauerkraut, kombucha, other fermented foods, and pro-biotics.

5. Exercise: It is now known that oxygen is essential in pre-venting and curing cancer. Hyperbaric oxygen, ozone, hyper-thermia, nitric oxide supplements, and physical exercise are all very beneficial for preventing and curing cancer. Dr. Budwig's muesli (flaxseed oil and cottage cheese or Quark, causes the body to produce high amounts of natural oxygen.

6. Believe that God will help you, and keep you healthy. This is very important in preventing and curing cancer. Dr. William Kelley, who cured his pancreatic cancer after oncologists had given him two months to live, said that his faith in God is what helped him cure his cancer. Faith in God is paramount in curing cancer.

7

The Greatest Medical Hoax in U.S. History

Have you ever wondered why American citizens in the U.S. pay four to five times more for medical treatment than people in all other countries? What is the reason for our high medical costs? When did this situation and medical hoax begin? Why don't we have a definite cure for many diseases including cancer, diabetes, and high blood pressure? Where does all the money for medical treatment go? How did Big Pharma end up being our biggest and most expensive medical treatment system? These questions and more need many answers and solutions. Do we need to change the most expensive medical system in the world?

There is no doubt that we all need physicians and associates to treat our many ills and diseases. They do a great job for most of our life-saving treatment and medical ills. But something has gone wrong with many medical treatments, and drugs that are being given today, especially in treating cancer.

In the shadows a long time ago, a certain millionaire connived to develop and control our U.S. medical system. From the very beginning, he developed a plan to start a system that ended up being Big Pharma, and the control of our medical, drug system, medical colleges, drug companies, and many doctors.

The following is hard to believe. Before 1878 most medical treatments in the U.S. were plant-based and physicians used homeopathic medicine. Almost all countries today use homeopathic treatment and plant-based medications. They not only surpass the U.S. in successful cures of cancer, diabetes, high blood pressure, and other diseases but have four to five times less cost for the patient.

We can trace the beginnings of Big Pharma to John D Rockefeller in 1878. He controlled a vast oil empire and made millions of dollars with over 80 percent of the oil business. Cars were just invented and the use of oil was just beginning.

His grandiose ideas in medicine and medical treatment came about in 1897 when the discovery of aspirin was made by Felix Hoffman, a German scientist. Rockefeller knew that a new medical frontier opened up with the use of petrochemicals. He visualized that petrochemicals could be the foundation for medicine including aspirin, penicillin, and other treatment drugs. Rockefeller realized that for him to expand his medical empire, he would have to change the plant-based homeopathic medicine, to a petrochemical medicine domination. This would be no small task.

First, he established the Rockefeller Institute for Medical Research. His leader, Fredrick Gates, in 1901, was influenced by a new book, "Principles and Practice of Medicine," written by Sir William Osler. Osler was an early pioneer of "Eugenics," The study of hereditary improvement by genetic control. What is interesting about this is that C.C. Little, a eugenics follower, and early president of the American Cancer Society, became the founding member of the Birth Control League, which eventually became known as Planned Parenthood.

In 1913, Rockefeller, his son, and Fredrick Gates joined in a new project. The goal was to justify the modernization, streamlining, and consolidation of medical teaching in medical schools and hospitals. The plan was to only offer grants and money to colleges that would go along with his patented based drug system. He gave out millions of dollars in grants, to the colleges that went along with his patented drug plan. This effort forced out most of the teaching for plant-based homeopathic medicine. This was a greedy, control effort that changed the course of medicine in the United States. Many homeopathic schools were closed, many hospitals had to change their direction from plant-based treatments. Some doctors were even jailed. This was the beginning of a new patented drug era, a pill for every ill.

After 1913, all medical schools and hospitals, scheduled to receive Rockefeller grants and money, were directed to teach and do research in directed medical areas, where these newly discovered drugs could be patented and sold in the many drug outlets within the Rockefeller empire. This included Squibb, which, at the time, was a wholly-owned Rockefeller business. Eventually, the drug companies underwrote the medical colleges, teaching the patented drug system

In 1938, the discovery of penicillin boosted Rockefeller's fortunes. During world war II, Big Pharma was well established and bringing in high profits. They were filtering money to the FDA, lobbyists, drug companies, and even cancer doctors. Over the past many years, Big Pharma has entrenched itself into the ropes of the government, FDA, lobbyists, drug companies, and doctors. Also, many of the smaller drug companies were bought out by the larger firms.

Researchers say that more than 50 percent of all Americans are over medicated. The Rockefeller dream has cost the U.S. patients billions of dollars. It has increased the insurance company's medical charges and profits over billions of dollars. Now, medical treatments and drugs cost American patients over 500 billion dollars a year, 200 billion for cancer alone.

But there is some hope. New technical research, artificial intelligence, cannabinoids, plant, and homeopathic medicines have begun to find many new treatment modalities, and alternative functional, and homeopathic medicine is on the rise. Hopefully, we may see some changes soon.

8

The Cause, Prevention, and Curing of Cancer

Part I

Since Otto Warburg discovered the cause of cancer in 1923, the disease has caused the death of millions of people all over the world. The United States usually has been the nation that leads to curing most diseases. However, in the case of cancer, and cancer research, about 90 percent of the money donated for research goes to the big drug companies for their patented drug research. If the treatment involves a non patented remedy, then the FDA, drug companies, and the medical establishment will not sanction or promote it in most cases. They will not promote a substance, or treatment, if it is not profitable to the drug companies, FDA (through kickbacks), and the medical establishment. Any homeopathic or other treatments are cast by the wayside.

Such is the case for the newer CellSonic electrohydraulic therapy machine and the 4 in 1 therapy machine. The CellSonic therapy machine sends high energy pulses into the cancer area, which changes the resonance and polarity of the cancer cells, and converts them back into the normal body, and organ cells. It is used in many countries to cure cancer, but not in the U.S. The 4 in 1 therapy machine utilizes hyperthermia and 3 other modalities to treat cancer. It also is showing some great advances in successful cancer treatment. Yet the FDA has yet to OK their use in the United States. You can learn more about the CellSonic therapy machine in Chapter 12. The Budwig cancer clinic in Spain has been using both the CellSonic and the 4 in 1 therapy machines for some time. Information can be obtained on their website.

Foreign nations are now leading the way in research and treatments in curing cancer with their homeopathic treatments, hyperthermia, I.V. vitamin C, mistletoe, 4 in 1 Therapy, and electric pulse therapy.

In the United States, new alternative cancer research, and the homeopathic treatment system have been on vacation for the last 70 years. Mostly, the U. S. customary cancer treatment consists of chemotherapy, radiation, surgery, and chemo drugs.

Recent research has brought about some very good changes in the cause and cure of cancer. Otto Warburg was the first man that showed us how the diet, an acid body, omega 6 oils, sugar, and carbohydrate consumption, with other contaminants and toxins, changed the chemical structure of the RNA (ribonucleic acid) and DNA (diribonucleic acid) inside the mitochondria of a body cell, which changed the polarity and started a cancer cell "hit." That is the start of cancer.

What are the factors in the body which lead up to the cancer cell "hit?" I will try to explain Otto Warburg's path to cancer, so you will be able to understand. The beginning usually starts with a person's diet. It involves the electrical structures of atoms. Ionic atoms are negative atoms, while cationic atoms are positive atoms. They make up the body cells, blood, and organs. Our bodies need more negative (anionic) atoms (made from raw live fresh foods). These anionic atoms create the energy that our bodies use. The cationic atoms are atoms that are positively charged atoms. They are made from foods that have very little or no electric charge. Cationic atoms are made from sugars, refined and processed carbohydrates, omega 6 (dead) oils which are on the grocery shelf, red meat fats, and other altered foods. Both anionic and cationic charged atoms are needed to produce electric charges. Together, they produce the energy that is needed in our intestinal flora, body cells, blood, and organs. However, we need more anionic body cells (from raw, fresh veggies, fruits, nuts, melons, berries, squash, leaves, etc.), than cationic body cells. When we eat more foods like sugar, carbohydrates, omega-six oils, refined and processed foods, etc., our bodies get acidic. Our body cells then get LESS ELECTRICAL CURRENTS, decreased energy, toxins, inflammation in the small intestine, and leaky gut. Disease creeps through the holes in the small intestine into the blood, causing disease.

These electromagnetic electric charges are measured by the pH, or acid/base balance. When we eat a high electrical charged diet, our bodies stay more healthy, our immune system is healthier, plus our body cells get more oxygen, plus more energy. These are the conditions that lead to good body cell pH, high energy, high electrical body cell, and immune system health.

Other conditions lead into the cationic low non-electromagnetic (pH), acetic, bad diet, mentioned above. This diet creates bad bacteria, candida fungus, and other bad organisms in the gut, which produce many toxins and intestinal inflammation. These conditions also produce a lower resonance and electrical body cell charge. The lower electrical impulses in acetic body cells (from acetic cationic diet) can change the chemical makeup of the DNA and RNA (amino acids) in the atoms (mitochondria), of an individual body cell, blood, or organs. This can cause a mutation in that particular cell, causing a cancer cell "hit." This lowers the acidity of the body cells even more, which lowers the body cell oxygen while creating many toxins. The cancer cells start multiplying with fermentation (they do not use oxygen to multiply). Glucose and the cancer's enzymes create excess lactic acid, which lowers conductivity even more.

The cancer cells do not use oxygen to multiply. They use sugar, glucose, carbohydrates, red meat protein, other body cells, etc., in a process called "glycosylation." They love an acidic body with high sugar, omega 6 oils, and a carbohydrate diet. It also usually takes 36 months before cancer is detected in the body. That is one reason why it is so hard to cure.

There are many ways that new machines, alternative, and homeopathic methods will cure cancer. Cancer cells use a lower electrical charge to metastasize and mutate. Because of this low electrical charge, very important new findings are paving the way for electrical pulse machines to treat cancer. Cancer treatment in many other nations is now including ways to send these high voltage electrical pulses, to increase the electrical charge in cancer cells. These pulses change the polarity and electric charge of cancer cells, causing them to change into normal cells. This eliminates the cancer tumors. Two of these machines are the CellSonic electrohydraulic therapy machine, and the 4 in 1 Therapy machine, mentioned earlier.

Proof of the cancer cell electrical pulse theory exists in the fact that cancer cells will not survive if a person has an electrical alkaline pH of 7.4 or more. Raising the electrical cell voltage and pH is the action of these high voltage pulse machines. The amazing thing is that these high voltage pulse machines will change the polarity of many other disease cells. This paves the way for many diseases to be cured. Some of these diseases that can be cured are avascular necrosis, spinal necrosis, muscular atrophy, prostate cancer, Alzheimer's disease, enlarged prostate, nonhealing wounds, rheumatoid arthritis, kidney stones, gall stones, wound healing, liver cirrhosis, and many more.

Several other successful alternative cancer treatments include foods and supplements that increase the red blood cell efficiency and body oxygen. Once a person understands what causes cancer, with poor diet, omega 6 oils, low cancer cell electrical impulses, plus the oxygen deprivation that the cancer cells produce, it can be cured. It is also possible to use diets and supplements to increase the oxygen, enzyme supplementation, change the body pH, eliminate the bad bacterial toxins, inflammation in the gut, plus eliminate several factors that allow cancer cells to multiply. (See Chapter 39)

Cancer is now being cured in many nations. Many cancer clinics in foreign countries are doing these procedures to cure 85 to 90 percent of their cancer patients. The oncologists in the U.S., with their chemo, radiation, surgery, and chemo drugs are still struggling to get more than an average 7 percent cancer cure rate over 5 years. In some cancer areas, they are doing better. In Joanna Budwig's cancer clinic in Spain, they have a very high rate of success. They are using the CellSonic electrohydraulic therapy machine and the 4 in 1 therapy to help them cure malignancies. However, they also are using many other treatments needed to cure cancer. (See Chapter 39)

I will not name all of the steps needed to cure cancer in this chapter. However, I will list six steps now, with many more to follow in the next two chapters. The list will include several methods used by foreign nation clinics, physicians, and their methods of curing cancer. They have cured thousands of patients, even grade III and IV cancer with these 22+ methods. Below are the first six very important steps in preventing and curing cancer. If you follow these and the other 16+ steps, plus do not stray away from the treatments, you can cure cancer. There will be many more steps to follow in the next two chapters.

1A. Dr. Budwig's cottage cheese, flaxseed oil, quark, and crushed flaxseeds formula: In chapter 1, I listed the directions. Check with your closest health food store to order Quark. An organic Quark by the brand name ELLI is available in large grocery stores in the states. Quark is easily found all over Europe. Many people use kefir, but that will not produce the same results. Her clinic uses this formula EVERY day, for their cancer patients. I would suggest that for the PREVENTION of cancer, it may be wise to use it THREE to FIVE times each week. This combination will help unravel sticky (homocysteine) blood, so red blood cells can carry more oxygen. Dr. Budwig said that most cancer patients have (sticky) blood. This formula is also very effective to unravel coagulated blood in high blood pressure, heart disease, and diabetic patients. If you have cancer, do not skip this critical step, and the pancreatic enzymes.

1B. Pancreatic enzymes: Dr. William Kelley was given two to four months to live after being diagnosed with liver and pancreatic cancer. He contributes his being able to cure cancer to massive amounts of pancreatic enzymes, plus his faith in God. Pancreatic enzymes attack and destroy cancer cells of all kinds. Do not try to get rid of cancer without using pancreatic enzymes. I will tell the story of Dr. William Kelley in another chapter. These enzymes are one of the two most important and critical cancer fighters, along with Dr. Joanna Budwig's alpha helix carbon molecule, cottage cheese/flaxseed oil/quark/flaxseed mixture. Pancreatic enzymes can be obtained from www.collegehealthstores. com or by calling 817 458 9241. For stopping and preventing cancer, Wobenzym-N is a great enzyme, although they are not as good as solozyme enzymes. Wobenzym-N enzymes can be obtained from the internet. Every cancer patient should take 15 to 18 pancreatic enzymes, whether solozymes or Wobenzym-N, between meals, EVERY DAY.

2. Sugar: This is also very critical. A cancer patient should stop all consumption of sugar, sugar-containing foods, refined, processed flour products, and carbohydrates. Most carbohydrates change into glucose when digested. Cancer cells multiply by fermentation. They use no oxygen. They love sugar, glucose, carbohydrates, and protein. The pancreas also only has enough insulin to process about 4 ounces of sugar/glucose at one time. Most people consume way over the average consumption of sugar/glucose, per person, per day. This does not include the carbohydrate consumption, which turns into glucose. For the prevention of cancer, a person should limit themselves to all sugar, refined, and processed carbohydrate foods. You can substitute it xylitol, honey, fresh raw nuts, sourdough, and fermented foods.

3. Vegetable oils on the grocery shelves: All omega 6 oils on the grocery shelf except extra virgin olive oil, are boiled, have no electric current, and are cationic, dead oils. These vegetable oils are a large part of the coagulation, sticky blood, and oxygen deprivation, in many cancer and heart disease patients. This same combination of oils is the cause of heart disease, strokes, heart attacks, clots in the veins, and clotting problems in many diabetics.

A cancer patient should stay away from fried, deep-fried, and other vegetable cooking oils. Also skip many other foods such as Crisco, margarine, mayonnaise, and several salad dressings, which contain these oils. Cancer patients need to avoid these oils altogether. Deep-fried oils can cause an immediate spiking of the omega 6 to omega 3 ratios, which can initiate immediate clotting of the blood in heart disease and cancer patients. If cooking oil is needed, coconut, palm oil, or butter is a much better choice.

4. Fresh raw vegetables, fruits, nuts, berries, bulbs, roots, leaves, and berries. All cancer patients should get EITHER 2-4 glasses of these raw fresh juices each day and/or eat 8 to 11+ of these raw, fresh foods that are mentioned above. These foods carry vitamins, minerals, enzymes, minerals, and amino acids needed for every person, every day. They are an essential part of preventing and curing cancer. The Gerson clinic feeds their cancer patients many glasses of raw, fresh juices each day. They juice 10-20 gallons of vegetables. They feel it is essential for

curing cancer. Eight to eleven+ of these raw, fresh foods and raw fresh juices should be in the diets of all preventive cancer people, every day.

5. Avoid all GMO foods: People who have cancer, or who want to prevent cancer, should not eat any corn or soy products unless they are organic. Always buy organic vegetables, fruits, and other fresh grown products. Stay away from the product, roundup, crops sprayed with roundup, and other Monsanto products. Thirty nations in the world have banned GMO products.

6. Coffee enemas: If you have cancer, coffee enemas are very CRITICAL and essential, every day. Use only, organic coffee. Cancer cells produce an excessive amount of toxins and dead cells. The toxins cause many body cell deaths. The coffee enemas are not only needed to detoxify the large intestine and stressed liver, but also to clean out a toxin residue that accumulates on the inside of the large intestine. Dr. Nicolas Gonzalez, when the medical establishment questioned his use of coffee enemas on over 10,000 cancer patients, stated that Dr. William Kelley also mandated coffee enemas on over 20,000 cancer patients, with no ill effects. Dr. Gonzalez also recommended coffee enemas (organic coffee) to PREVENT cancer, using preventive coffee enemas once every 6 months or year. Both were very successful in curing cancer. Dr. Gonzalez also used coffee enemas to prevent cancer on himself with no ill effects. This is where a cancer MANAGER is very helpful.

There are many more critical and essential treatments people need to prevent and cure cancer. These treatments will be included in the next two chapters.

In foreign nations, 85 to 90 percent of the tumors in cancer patients are being cured with these homeopathic and alternative preventive cancer treatments, which include the use of coffee enemas. Also, in many foreign countries, cancer treatment centers are using voltage pulse machines, Dr. Budwig's formula, and Dr. Kelley's enzymes to cure cancer.

These are 7 of the 22 steps to cure cancer. All 22 steps are critical, and essential in curing cancer. Number one is in two Steps 1A and 1B because these are the two most critical steps for every cancer patient to take EVERY DAY. Every cancer patient must be taking these steps to cure cancer, whether they are taking chemo, radiation, or chemo drugs. They should be on every cancer victim's most critical list. Many more will be presented in my next two chapters. If you desire, it may be good to print the steps in Chapter 39, which is a complete list of all 23+ treatment steps.

9

The Cause, Prevention, and Curing Cancer

Part II

In the last Chapter, I covered how cancer cells get their start. Most cancers get their start because the immune system is weak. Dr. William Kelley, who cured himself of pancreatic cancer after the oncologist had given him only two to four months to live, stated; "Cancer starts in a sick body." Most people today have a weak, low electromagnetic immune system, from eating many cationic acidic foods, that lower the body pH (acid/base balance). This allows toxins, candida fungus, and even other parasites to weaken the immune system. In this chapter, I will expand on the prevention and cure for cancer.

The 22+ steps in these three chapters for curing cancer have been used all over the world by many alternative physicians in helping cure cancer. There are always risks in using alternative treatments to cure cancer. The same risks also exist in using the oncologist's treatment. Alternative treatments can be used with or without the oncologist's cancer treatment, or with lessor chemotherapy combined with alternative I.V. or other treatments. It is always wise to get your physician's or oncologist's advice before using any alternative or preventive treatment.

The results of cancer treatments may also vary from one individual to another. There is one axiom that all alternative physicians state. That if you have cancer, and use alternative treatment, you must adhere to the complete cancer treatment. That may be expensive, but not as expensive as the oncologist's treatment in most cases, or losing your life. If you smoke or drink excessively, do not change your diet to a neutral alkaline, non-acidic diet, do not use coffee enemas, or FOLLOW ALL of the 22+ instructions, you will be playing Russian roulette with your life. Your results may end in failure.

I mentioned sugar, sugared products, vegetable oils on the grocery shelf, and four other very important treatments that need to be followed, to prevent, and cure cancer. In this chapter, I will continue to cover several other very essential steps that a person must follow to prevent and treat cancer. They are very important and if possible, must be followed to prevent and/or cure cancer

7. Barley Powder: Barley powder is very critical as it is needed to raise the acidity of a cancer victim's body. However, a test should be made with litmus paper every day on your urine and saliva, to make sure that your body is not getting more alkaline than normal. Barley powder comes in powder form and capsules. Barley powder can be obtained at the health food store and can be used by putting one to three teaspoons of powder into soups and liquids during the day. Capsules can be obtained from "Green Supreme." A person can call 800 358 0777 or email www.GreenSupreme.net. I use both forms for prevention. If you have cancer and are taking the capsules, you may need to take 10 to 15 capsules a day if your urine and saliva are very acidic. If it is alkaline, you will not need to take much barley powder. You can check your pH with litmus paper.

8. Oral vitamin C, L-Proline, and L-Lycine: Do not skip this combination. Linus Pauling used these three ingredients to stop cancer cells in their tracks. He also used I.V. vitamin C to kill cancer cells. Without vitamin C, I.V., for prevention, take 2000 mg per day, and with cancer, 4,000 to 6,000 mg. vitamin C. However, please keep in mind that you should not do Vitamin C IV's at the same time you are consuming the flaxseed oil and cottage cheese/Quark muesli, otherwise these two remedies, used at the same time will clash with each other and you will nullify the benefits of both therapies. So if you are determined to have vitamin C infusions, wait until you finish those sessions, and then start to consume the Budwig muesli. Normal vitamin C dissolves rapidly in the blood, it disperses in about 2 to 3 hours, therefore it is best to take some at breakfast time and then again at noon. Be sure to only use natural vitamin C, such as acerola, not ascorbic acid.

9. Beta-1, 3D glucan: This supplement is an immune system booster. It goes into the bloodstream and is one of the best cancer cell destroyers, along with trypsin, and enzymes. It enhances the immune system in destroying cancer cells. A person can get the supplement by calling 855 877 8220 or on the website www.ancient5.com The dosage for cancer is 3 tabs daily, taken in the morning. .This is very essential for curing cancer.

10. Vegetable juice: The Gerson clinic feeds their cancer patients 4 to 5 glasses of raw, fresh juiced vegetable juice every day. WITH THIS cancer regime, a person with cancer might bring that down to 2 to 3 glasses. At any rate, it is great. One glass a day is great for prevention, two to three with cancer.

11. Red meat: With cancer, eat NO RED MEAT. Limit white meat to only small portions, two to three times a week. Cancer cells love sugar and PROTEIN. For prevention, a person should eat red meat sparingly. Substitute with raw almonds, pecans, and walnuts, and spirulina which contains more natural protein than meat.

12. Fenbendazole: Hulda Clark, in her great book, "The Cure for All Cancer," states that liver flukes and other parasites cause cancer. She said that 90 percent of all cancer patients have parasites. Therefore, I recommend all cancer patients, and all preventive cancer people, have a parasite cleanse once a year. Should you be able to get it, fenbendazole has rid many people of cancer. A book, written by Joe Tippens, describes his bout with cancer. His cancer had metastasized to all parts of his body. His oncologist gave him only a few months to live. But Joe was not one to give up. He had a veterinarian friend who suggested fenbendazole, which is used to eliminate parasites in dogs. Joe started taking the measured amount for his weight. He also changed his diet and did many things listed in my cancer bulletins. Joe's cancer was gone in three months. Since that time, from Joes suggestions, many other cancer patients have used fenbendazole to cure their cancer. If you cannot find fenbendazole, a good parasite cleanser can be found on the internet called "Purify." You can contact www.thelifetree.com. Dr. Hulda Clarke's store also has a parasite cleanser, "intestinal edge." It can be found on her website.

13. Vitamin D3, Turmeric, Gingko Biloba, L-arginine, and L-gluta-mine: These supplements are very important for creating nitrous oxide, and oxygen in the body. With cancer, vitamin D3 (also great for coro-navirus), is very important for fighting cancer. A cancer patient needs to take about 25, 000 I.U. of D3 each day for 4 to 5 weeks. Then it can be reduced to 10,000 I.U.s per day. With the other supplements above, you can follow the recommended dosages.

14. Dr. Budwig had all of her patients lying in the sun for 10 minutes on the front and then 10 minutes on the back of the body with as much skin exposed as possible for several minutes for natural vitamin D. For prevention, these supplements are as important as when a person has cancer.

15. Root Canals: Almost all alternative and preventative cancer phy-sicians recommend that cancer patients have their root canal teeth ex-tracted. Most of the older root canals have been proven to be non-ster-ile. In preventing cancer, I would not recommend removal. With cancer, it would be a good choice.

16. Insula Peptide: Peptide supplements, formed by a combination of amino acids, are being used as a new approach to curing cancer nat-urally. Peptides, including insula peptide, is widely used in Mexico as a safe cancer therapy. Peptides are related to enzymes and are very essential in cancer treatment. If they would use amino acids and pep-tides, oncologists would only need small amounts of chemo drugs to destroy large amounts of cancer cells. However, most U.S. oncologists refrain from using enzymes and peptides., even though they are very effective. Mexican physicians are using insula peptide in many cases, with a great result. You can get peptides from New England Peptides, 1 800 343 5974.

17. Dr. Joanna Budwig's cancer clinic: Dr. Budwig has made a tremen-dous contribution to cancer treatment all over the world. She discov-ered the cottage cheese/ flaxseed oil combination which uses the alpha helix carbon molecule to unravel sticky blood. She treated 2,500 grade III and IV cancer patients with an 85 to 90 percent successful living rate over 5 years. Her cancer clinic in Spain still treats cancer patients (with great success) today. The cancer clinic's new addition of the Cell-

Sonic electrohydraulic therapy machine, and the 4 in 1 therapy, have also been a great contribution to their success. They plan to open a clinic in Florida and have the 4 in one therapy machine. They are applying to use it for cancer therapy. They are using the therapy in many other ways also. It can treat many diseases with a very good success rate. If you, your relative, friend, or neighbor has cancer, access to the Arizona facility, and the manager, Dr. Lloyd Jenkins, can be reached by email at PlanetBudwig@gmail.com. or the Budwig website, www. BudwigCenter.com

There are more essential cancer therapies that will be included in the next chapter. As I said before, if a person has cancer, it will be very critical and essential to follow all of these steps to eradicate this disease. For people who want to PREVENT cancer, I have not listed many of the dosages. You will need to look up some of them. Believe me, all of these steps are very important for curing cancer, and preventing cancer.

It is also very important to get a cancer manager, to help you. A cancer manager, spouse, friend, or relative can help you with enemas, buying the supplements, help you with dosages, and ordering products. This is very serious and is a critical and essential part of cancer treatment.

The future of preventing and curing cancer has a lot of promise. Artificial Intelligence will give people the opportunity for many new cancer tests and therapies. An exciting cancer cure future awaits.

10

The Cause, Prevention, and Cure for Cancer

Part III

Cancer is a very stress full disease. But it is not a disease that a person cannot overcome. With the right diet, the right treatments, the right determination, and help from God, a person will have the right recipe to overcome all odds. By following the twenty-two plus treatment guides listed in these three chapters, and chapter 39, many thousands have cured cancer. Many studies have shown that a great attitude, a great social environment, a great cancer program, a great cancer manager, and faith in God, have cured thousands of cancer patients. God has given us the tools to cure cancer. We need to be vigilant, follow the steps, and not miss any unless it is impossible to get or do. PLEASE do not miss any of the steps.

Do not think that curing cancer is an easy task. A person has to spend 100 percent of their time working to cure cancer. They have to follow the treatments, 100 percent, and they have to be determined to win. They have to have a good manager. Win they can do when they have faith in God, are 100 percent dedicated, and follow these 22+ treatment steps. REMEMBER, a cancer manager is CRITICAL.

Many things are a great help. One is to reduce stress as much as possible. Many alternative cancer physicians have stated clearly that bad emotions, stress, negative thinking, and depression are very damaging for cancer patients. People that are very happy, and have a great social life, have a lot less cancer than those who are stressed, depressed, have many of life's troubles, or think negatively. These factors bring to mind the words of Mahatma Gandhi, which make good sense when a person has cancer. "Men often become what they believe themselves to be. If they believe they cannot do something, it makes them incapable of doing it. But when they believe they can, then they will acquire the ability to succeed, even though they do not have the ability in the beginning."

I'm sure God believes in the same quotation. If a person believes in him, he will be with them through their cancer journey. With his help, you will believe you will overcome cancer, and you can do it.

This final cancer prevention and cure chapter will list the last additional steps in cancer treatment. These are also very important recommendations for preventing and curing cancer. These 22+ cancer cure treatments are the result of three years of research and searching through over a half dozen cancer clinics, plus several alternative U.S. and foreign homeopathic physician's successful cancer treatment. It also involves information in many books on curing cancer. The abbreviated steps are also in chapter 39.

18. The Sauna and/or hot baths: The cancer treatment in many cancer clinics include using the sauna or hot baths every day. Cancer cells cannot live at a pH of 7.4 or higher. They also are not able to live with high body temperatures over 108 degrees Fahrenheit. High temperatures over 100 degrees will SUPPRESS the spread of cancer cells. That is why the sauna and/ or hot baths are a great cancer cell treatment. This creates a rise in body temperature which weakens and even kills some cancer cells. It also improves circulation. Another plus is that it also helps remove toxins from a person's body. Saunas can be found in most U.S. cities. If a cancer victim cannot find a sauna, then 102-104 degree hot baths, for 45 minutes, to an hour daily, would be a good substitute.

19. Apricot seeds and laetrile: Many physicians in Mexico use I.V. laetrile to treat cancer, along with other modalities. Many alternative and preventative cancer physicians in the U.S. use another approach. They go to the source, apricot seeds. They state that 12 to 15 apricot seeds, eaten throughout the day, are a great cancer cell destroyer. Apricot seeds can be obtained by checking chapter 39. The source will be listed there. A great laetrile product called "Amygdalina," can be obtained in a Mexican pharmacy online, or by email; www.cytopharmaonline. com, or call 1 888 271 4184. If they do not have laetrile, they will know

where to get it. More information can be obtained on a website named; www.apricotpower.com

20. Mercury fillings: Many people do not realize this, but what the ADA and many dentists call, "silver fillings," have about 50 percent mercury. Most dentists have stopped using amalgam (silver-mercury) fillings. Mercury fillings produce vapors that even are present when a person grinds on a mercury filling for weeks, months, and even years later. To prevent cancer, a person would be wise to eliminate any mercury fillings. To cure cancer, many alternative cancer physicians recommend the cancer patient have their amalgam fillings replaced. There are several protective procedures used by dentists who are replacing amalgam fillings. If a person has them removed, they should have the procedure done by a dentist trained in amalgam removal.

21. pH testing: Any person serious about preventing or curing cancer, would be wise to buy and use roll type oral hydrion litmus paper. The ranges that a person needs are 4.5 pH to 8.5 or 9.0 pH. It can be gotten from health food stores, online, Daily manufacturing, or see chapter 39. Be sure that it is in rolls and used for urine and saliva testing. A person preventing cancer, or having cancer should take their urine and saliva pH every morning when they get up and every evening before they brush their teeth and go to bed. The ideal urine and body pH is 6.4. That is when all of the body systems are running great and your blood and the immune system are very good. Readings of 6.2 to 6.8, mean that your acid/base balance is good. When the readings are under 6.2, acidic (yellow), or 6.8, alkaline (blue), then the diet needs to be corrected to adjust for a neutral acid/alkaline balance. I have mentioned before the foods necessary to bring an acidic pH up, and what foods are needed to bring an alkaline pH down. More information can be obtained by looking at the websites online for Dr. A.F. Beddoe, and Dr. Carey Reams.

22. Microwaved foods: When a person puts any food in the microwave. It nukes the food. Microwaved food has no electromagnetic charge. That means it does not contribute to energy, health, and longevity. Many Mexican restaurants microwave their food. It is best to use the oven when heating foods up. If the heat is not over 350 degrees, and the

food is not left in the oven for over 10-12 minutes, some electromagnetic value may still be present.

23. Garlic: I wanted to mention fresh, raw garlic again. It is very valuable to a person's health. Every day, a person would be wise to crush or finely chop 3-5 garlic cloves and put them in their food. Now you can enjoy black fermented garlic, as it provides more health benefits and you have no garlic breath or odor as with regular garlic. Do not use so many cloves that the taste is bitter. Crushing releases the allicin, which has tremendous benefits for a person's health. Garlic does a great many great things for the immune system, prevention of cancer, plus has many antibiotic properties. It is surely a great food and is one of the most important foods a person can eat.

These twenty-two preventive and cancer-curing treatments are the culmination of three years of research. These procedures, foods, and treatments, have prevented and helped cure over 200,000+ people all over the world, with cancer. This may be a long list of things to do, but they work with almost all cancer patients. Even in combination with conventional treatment with chemo, radiation, and chemo drugs, they would be a great help in curing cancer. For PREVENTING cancer, this is a great benefit, although the dosages, times, and recommendations need to be adjusted. I have not adjusted the dosages for prevention in many cases. and a person needs to do a little research to find information about the dosages.

These are also not medical treatments. Any person using these procedures, or treatments, should get the advice of their physician or oncologist before using this information.

11

25+ Trillion Electromagnetic Engines in the Small Intestine

That's right, each cell in your body is a tiny electromagnetic engine, and it runs on tiny electromagnetic impulses called "Hertz" or "pH." pH = acid – NEUTRAL– Alkaline." Neutral pH (6.4) is the best impulse or electromagnetic charge to keep your body cells and organs healthy. Your body can get acidic, or alkaline. Both can cause a disease state. But an alkaline state is not as bad as having acidic, low urine, saliva, body cell, and blood pH. Your car has one electric motor. It also runs on electric impulses from the battery or generator, called "volts." An electric short will stop the engine. The car is then dead in the water. There is a big advantage for humans to have trillions of electric motors.

Thousands of your tiny body cell engines can get shorted out, and you can still function. Surgeons take out prostate glands, appendix, breasts, and many other organs, without a total short, because unlike the car, the other engines in the body can keep it running. When you have a disease or blood clot, it shorts out those particular body cells, but in most cases, other cells can keep the other 2.5+ trillion intestinal bacteria and body cells functioning.

Human cells function because of the electromagnetic energy gotten from live plant foods. Minerals, vitamins, enzymes, amino acids, and other nutrients are obtained from the soil in the roots of plants and they provide electromagnetic energy.

Toxins and inflammation from bad bacteria, candida fungus. viruses, and parasite larvae short out millions of body cells. The toxins, candida, bad bacteria, and parasite larvae go through holes in the small intestine (leaky gut) and cause disease. However, with 2.5+ trillion cells, thousands of them can be shorted out and the body will still function, but not on optimum levels. To stay healthy, your job is to eat good foods that prevent electromagnetic shorting, and the death of body cells. The better the diet with electromagnetic foods, the better the health of your body, the less disease, and cancer.

All body cells are important but red, and white blood cells are extremely important. They carry the fuel (oxygen, vitamins, minerals, enzymes, and other nutrients) that carry the energy and electromagnetic impulses.

Toxins and inflammation from bad foods (refined foods, processed foods, sugar, omega 6 oils, etc.) short out the red blood cells (they then can produce homocysteine, a clotting factor) and they become sticky. Sticky blood causes strokes, heart attacks, and blood clots in diabetes, and cancer.

Dr. Linus Pauling discovered the double carbon bond helix molecule. These are the most electromagnetic molecules in the human body. Double bond helix molecule substances will unravel sticky blood.

Dr. Joanna Budwig, a biochemist, found how to create the double bond helix molecules, which can unravel sticky (homocysteine) blood. By the way, over 35 percent of people in the U.S., eat a bad diet and have high blood pressure, which can cause sticky blood (see the cover, and page 3). Dr. Budwig created a cottage cheese, flaxseed oil mixture that can prevent and unravel sticky blood. This enables the red blood cells to carry more oxygen, especially needed to prevent cancer. In most cancer patients, cancer cells create homocysteine or sticky blood. Oxygen is the other great propellent for helping destroy cancer cells. Cancer cells want no oxygen since they multiply by a process with the sugar called glycolysis or glycosylation. Oxygen helps get rid of cancer cells.

Why is the double helix bond molecule so important? It is a formula that Dr. Budwig used, which separates sticky blood, so it can carry more OXYGEN. Her formula should be eaten daily, with every cancer person's breakfast diet, and/or a preventive cancer person's diet, three to seven times a week. What is the formula that Dr. Budwig discovered? Four ingredients are needed. 1. Low fat 2% or less cottage cheese or Quark, 6 tablespoons. 2. Flaxseed oil, 4 tablespoons. 3. 1 teaspoon of raw honey, and if the mixture is very dry, 2 tablespoons of low-fat milk. Mix with an electric mixer if possible. Add to mixture. 4. Flax-seeds, (two-level tablespoon's) grind in coffee bean mixer. For taste, berries, pineapple, or fruit can be added.

This mixture was the main part of the diet, plus several other procedures, which helped cure 85 % of 2,500+ grade III and grade IV cancer patients in Germany at Dr. Budwig's hospital.

Going back to the 25+ trillion body cells, they need raw fresh vegetables, fruits, melons, berries, roots, nuts, protein, eggs, and leaves plus polyunsaturated oils to create electromagnetic energy to fuel the body cells.

Shorting out our millions of body cells and organs with bad foods and oils will sometimes short out cells and organs until the important ones will quit working. If too many body cells short out, the person gets to the same point as the car and its battery. The total body engine will not start.

In a cancer book that I read, one person that treats cancer patients has been eating Dr. Budwig's formula for twelve years. He has never even had a cold. My wife and I have been using it for two years, 3 to 5 times a week. We are planning on using Dr. Budwig's formula for the rest of our lives.

12

The New CellSonic VIPP Machine

Very Intense Pressure Pulses

Very recently, a new cancer treatment therapy machine was introduced into the cancer treatment world. The Budwig Center in Spain uses this machine in the cancer clinic and is obtaining remarkable results in a very short time. It is called the CellSonic VIPP machine. (Very Intense Pressure Pulses) If you, a friend, relative, or neighbor has cancer or many other diseases, it may be a wise decision to look into this new, revolutionary machine.

What is the CellSonic VIPP machine? I have mentioned many times that every cell in the body has a positive (ionic) and a negative (cationic) electric charge. There is a weakening of the resonance, and electric charges in cancer and many other disease cells. This means that many diseases have a weakened or lower electrical charge. This CellSonic cancer therapy machine switches the weak polarity of cancer, and other disease cells back into the correct alignment.

It works with a process of medical electrical pressure pulses that provoke the cancer cells. The pulses are generated by a sonic bang when the high voltages of the machine are directed by a hand pointer into the cancer cell area. The voltages of the machine are adjustable, depending on whether it is treating cancer, kidney stones, gall stones, rheumatoid arthritis, or many other diseases that it can treat. The machine changes the POLARITY of the cancer cells into alignment. The remarkable result is that when the cancer cells multiply, instead of replicating into more cancer cells they change into regular, healthy normal body cells. The intense pressure pulse that the machine produces changes the mutated cells, increases vascular cells, repairs nerves, and stops the tumor. It heals without any collateral damage to the surrounding tissues.

Professor Andrew Hague, president of CellSonic corporation, has said that for many cancers, including prostate and breast cancer, the machine has been very successful. Several thousand cancer patients have now been treated in Mexico, Switzerland, Spain, India, Poland, Germany, Peru and over 14 other countries. All of the practitioners have had the same successful results, not only with one type but with several types of cancers. Also, in many types of cancers, remarkable success has been seen with other diseases and ailments, including gall stones, kidney stones, sports injuries, wound healing, rheumatic arthritis, migraine headaches, enlarged prostates, stenosis, avascular necrosis, diabetes, TMJ disorders, cellulite, wrinkles, and many other conditions. The machine has different energy adjustments for each corresponding disease or ailment. The treatments are patient-friendly, with no invasive changes, or side effects at all.

Professionals who use the CellSonic machine have claimed that they have had success treating ALL TYPES of CANCER, plus many other diseases. It is simple to use with adjustments and a handheld applicator which is used with a gel on the skin. One advantage of the CellSonic therapy machine is that even in grade III and IV cancers, there has been a rapid decrease in the changing of the cancer cells. Many patients claimed that by the fourth day of treatment, they could feel the increased wellness.

Using the CellSonic machine is very easy. The preparation of the skin and area is the same as for any other medical procedure. It takes only a few minutes to perform the treatment. The simple instructions that are sent with the machine explain that the treatment can be done by a locally trained nurse.

The doctors at the Budwig Cancer clinic in Spain, CAUTION that there are MANY OTHER TREATMENT THERAPIES are needed to cure cancer, besides the CellSonic machine therapy. After the tumor has been stopped, the healing of the damage caused, begins.

The protocol is to correct the patient's diet including the elimination of toxins with coffee and garlic enemas, the Budwig cottage cheese (or quark) formula, twice a day, enzyme therapy, fermented foods, sunlight, hyperthermia, Four in 1 infrared therapy. along with plant-based herbal supplements. Cancer patients also need to stop all sugars, sugar substances, refined and processed carbohydrates, red meat, (Dr. Budwig says no meat), and no omega 6 oils (gotten from the grocery shelf), etc.

Patients undergoing chemotherapy, radiation, and, or chemo drugs are cautioned to wait four weeks before beginning CellSonic treatment. They also need to continue the cancer diet, toxic elimination supplements, enzyme therapy, and other cancer regimes.

With FDA approval, patients living in Canada and the U.S. will have the opportunity for a reasonably priced cancer treatment by emailing Dr. Lloyd Jenkins at PlanetBudwig@gmail.com. This treatment is an option that cancer patients may explore for their cancer treatment. It seems to be very promising.

We are hoping that someday soon this machine will be approved by the FDA for use in the U.S., and Canada.

CELLSONIC & BUDWIG PROTOCOL

CLINICAL STUDIES – TESTEMONIALS

Dolores Garcia Rodriquez

Abdominal Cancer: Stage 3 – Cancer Markers CA125 at 566 U/ml

Feb 26, 2020, came to Budwig Center for CellSonic sessions. Cancer markers CA125 dropped from 566 to 348 which is 218 units lower after one short session over the stomach only and one complete session over all the major organs and spinal column.

Translation: The Oncologist that we saw yesterday examined the stomach tumor and stated that it is smaller and not as hard as before, but softer. He said he had never heard of hyperthermia nor CellSonic and the other treatments"

The Budwig Center has given Dolores the Budwig dietary recommendations and some specific anti-cancer remedies and she will return in 2 months for more treatment.

Annalina Malachia

Stage 2 Left Breast Cancer – 2 lumps 13 and 14 mm

Feb 24, 2020, came to Budwig Center and received CellSonic treatment as well as all the major organs and spinal column. She received hyperthermia whole body, Four in One therapy, Magnetic therapy, lymphatic drainage, emotional rebalancing, and followed the Budwig food plan and supplements for 2 weeks.

CA-15.3 Cancer Marker test March 5, 2020 – 30 or more indicates Cancer

Colin Weatherly

Aggressive Prostate Cancer PSA 15

Started treatment at the Budwig Center on Feb 24, 2020, and received 2 sessions of CellSonic over the prostate, as well as all the major organs and spinal column. Colin received hyperthermia whole body, Four in One therapy, Magnetic therapy and followed the Budwig food plan and supplements.

PSA dropped from 15 to 12,6 after just 2 weeks. Colin will continue now on the full Budwig protocol and normally when cancer markers start to go down if the patients stay on the Budwig plan, they continue to decrease until cancer no longer shows up on the tests. Clinical bio-resonance tests also show remarkable improvements.

Ellen (Anja) Kirschawn

Liver Cancer and back and neck pain level 8

Started treatment at the Budwig Center on Feb. 24, 2020, and received CellSonic over the liver, as well as all the major organs and spinal column.

Ellen received hyperthermia whole body, Four in One therapy, Magnetic therapy, emotional rebalancing and followed the Budwig food plan and supplements for 3 weeks. She no longer complains of any pain and the echo graph from Vithas hospital shows no cancer activity. She also received clinical bio-resonance tests with Zyto and VEGA test show remarkable improvements.

13

Many Cancers are Most Likely Caused by Sugar and Carbs

To prevent or cure cancer, sugar is one of the most important, paramount things to eliminate from your diet. Ingesting sugar when you want to prevent, or have cancer, is like pouring gasoline on a fire. Sugar is an enemy to your health and does more harm to your body than even tobacco and alcohol. Excess refined sugar, sugar products, and carbohydrates produce an insulin release, using up insulin, and depriving the pancreas of producing other enzymes that help prevent and destroy cancer.

The average consumption of sugar products per person/year, in the U.S., is 120 lbs. That is averaging about 22 teaspoons/day for every single person in the U.S. What one doesn't think about is that most carbohydrates also turn to sugar in the body, by a process called glycation. Pasta, bread, potatoes, pizzas, and noodles are in that group. I'm saying that it would be good to eat carbohydrates, but it is good to limit them and if eating them, use whole grain flour in carbohydrate foods. White flour has no nutrients as all. The nutrients are in the husks. Pizzas, pastries, donuts, bread, and potatoes. William Kelley stated: to prevent cancer, "limit carbs." With cancer, they should be eliminated. When people have cancer, Dr. William Kelley stated; "limit carbs to almost zero."

Most of the sugars that a person ingests are in the form of fructose (HFCS) and corn syrup (HFCS). These are found in more and more refined foods. People can get addicted to sugar, corn syrup, and fructose. Retailers use this to their advantage. Also, most refined sugar is made from GMO sugar beets.

American children are consuming ten times more sugar and sugar products than they were consuming 40 years ago. Eating excess GMO sugar, fructose, and corn syrup will lead to acetic problems in the children's, and adult's cells, organs, and immune system. Diabetes and obesity have been diagnosed in over 35 percent of the population.

Cancer cells use 20 times more sugar than normal cells, so when a person has a sugar diet, cancer cells are more likely to form, and if so, they are in their glory. Once a person has cancer, without completely stopping sugar and carbohydrate consumption, it is almost impossible to prevent or to stop cancer cells. If you research the foods with hidden sugar, you will find it is incredible. These are some of the foods that have sugar or fructose (HFCS): Ice cream, ketchup, mayonnaise, 60% of all refined foods, salad dressing, pastries, sodas, most power drinks, most ham, many sausages. many kinds of bread and cereals, 95% of deserts, many energy drinks, plus many more foods.

Most important also, is to reduce all carbohydrates. Cancer cells love bread, pasta, macaroni, noodles, crackers, breakfast cereals, potatoes, white flour, white rice, and many other carbohydrates. Most of these carbohydrates convert to sugar in the body. All of these sugars and substitutes need to be reduced or eaten sparingly to prevent or eradicate cancer. Cancer cells use no oxygen and reproduce with sugar.

Ingesting a high sugar and carbohydrate diet will cause white blood cells, (macrophages, leucocytes, monocytes, lymphocytes, eosinophils, basophils, and neutrophils) to drop dramatically. As I mentioned before, cancer cells are resistant to these immune cells, because they produce a protein masking substance that mimics regular cells.

This lowering of the immune system allows the patient to get other diseases like pneumonia, allergies, intestinal colitis, Crohn's disease, and many other diseases. Most cancer patients do not die from cancer, but by the ailments, gotten because the immune system is so deficient, it cannot get rid of the toxins and side diseases. Sugar molecules attach to proteins and aid in the growth of cancer itself. Removal of high fructose corn syrup (HFCS), fructose, and refined sugars are now proven to have an enormous impact on preventing, and/or curing cancer.

Eliminate all sugar substitutes, except xylitol, coconut, and limited honey. Sugar substitutes, not counting honey, coconut, and xylitol, are worse than sugar when it comes to treating cancer. One physician stated that diet sodas were the number one worst food in the nation. To prevent, or if one is treating cancer, please stay away from most sugar substitutes. 90% of all corn syrup and fructose is made from GMO corn unless it is organic. Unless otherwise stated on the label, HFCS is found in most refined foods. If sugar isn't bad enough, corn syrup and fructose are GMO modified (genetically modified) food made from GMO sugar beets and corn. In 2008 the FDA deregulated sugar and fructose, allowing GMO sugars to be sold in the United States without putting anything on the labels. In most countries, GMO products are prohibited.

Since GMO corn syrup (HFCS) and fructose are very inexpensive, they are used almost 100 percent of the time in pastries, refined foods, mayonnaise, ketchup, salad dressing, and almost all foods that use sweets. Artificial sweets, plus other sugar substitutes should not be used when preventing or arresting cancer. They are more harmful than sugar, fructose, and HFCS.

14

The Silent Cancer and Heart Disease Killer:
Sticky Blood

What is sticky blood? It is a condition in your arteries and veins related to your red blood cells. The free separated red blood cells can be changed by a person's diet to form sticky, coagulated red blood cells. The results can be very detrimental to a person's health. (see the book cover and page 3)

There are two commonly related blood clot diseases. Sticky blood platelet disease, and homocysteine related red blood cell inflammation, which will also cause blood disease. The red blood cell homocysteine is related to poor diet, excess sugar consumption, omega 6 oils from off the grocery shelf, refined, processed foods, and excess red meat. In many cases, the homocysteine in a person's blood can be associated with diabetes, heart disease, and cancer. This is logical because many diabetic patients also have homocysteine in their blood. A result of excess sugar, and insufficient insulin in body cells. Research has shown that folate, folic acid, vitamin B6, and B12 will reduce homocysteine in the blood. People with kidney disease or kidney failure need to be aware that large dosages of these vitamins are harmful and not recommended for renal impairment patients.

Homocysteine is an amino acid that is biosynthesized from methionine. A high concentration of it in the blood can cause inflammation of the red blood cells leading to clotting of the blood. It is a negative factor in diabetes and heart disease. Diabetes is a high cause of clotting in the eyes, brain, arteries, and veins in the legs. Clotting of the legs is the reason why some people lose their limbs. Diabetics can also lose their vision.

A regular blood test will not usually detect homocysteine. However, a good test is the glycated hemoglobin test. The normal glycated hemoglobin range should be 5 to 5.5. A range of 6 to 6.5 percent is associated with about 10 times more risk for diabetes, heart attack, stroke, and cancer. It is a shame that more physicians do not use this test.

The formation of homocysteine in cancer leads to a very interesting and exciting story. After Linus Pauling and two other Nobel prize winners found the double helix bond carbon molecule, Dr. JoAnna Budwig found that about 80 percent of cancer patients had homocysteine in their blood. The German biochemist also discovered a mixture that would unwind homocysteine blood in cancer patients. She discovered a special ingredient mix, that formed a double helix bond. The process would free the sticky blood so the red blood cells would carry more oxygen.

Dr. Budwig started treating grade III and IV cancer patients after they were dismissed from the regular cancer doctor's unsuccessful treatment with chemotherapy and radiation. They were given a short time to live. She had her hospital treat over 2,500 grade III and grade IV cancer patients. With her cottage cheese formula and many other procedures, she started having an 85 to 90 percent success rate in curing these dismissed cancer patients. She also used several other procedures with supplements, sauna, sunlight, pulse instruments, vitamins, and fresh raw foods in her treatment. Soon, other cancer clinics in Germany started using the same mixture, and procedures with great success.

Although Dr. Budwig is deceased, her cancer clinic treats cancer patients today in Spain, which you can check on her website, or with google. Her clinic recommends this cottage cheese/flaxseed/kefir combination for their patients one to two times daily. For a person who wants to prevent diabetes, cancer, or high blood pressure, this is a great combination to use 3 – 5 times each week.

If you are being treated for cancer, and your oncologist does not want you to use this mixture, he is not giving you the best recommendation for your health. If you have an alternative or functional medicine physician, I am sure they would welcome your dietary suggestion.

One of the worst causes of homocysteine is eating fried or deep-fried chicken, potatoes (French fries), fish, and hamburgers in Omega 6 oils, which are bought on the grocery shelf. Canola and corn oils (GMO products) are two of the worst culprits. Also, many restaurants use these oils over and over. These oils are non-electromagnetic dead oils and harm your health. They are also the biggest factor in homocysteine formation. If you want to fry any food, using coconut oil, palm oil, or butter is a much better choice.

15

The FDA, National Cancer Institute, and the Oncologists

The National Cancer Institute (NCI) is part of the National Institute of Health. The Institute of Health is one of the eleven agencies that are part of the U.S. Department of Human Services. The NCI was established in 1937 and has two research labs participating in research on cancer drugs. It was added to the Department of Health and Welfare in 1944, 75 years ago.

Since the NCI was established, it has only performed research on patented cancer drugs. It has also sponsored drug companies that were doing research, mostly petrochemical cancer drugs, and ones that can be patented. In the last 75 years, it has not done any research on the cause of cancer, plant-based drugs, or alternative homeopathic drug treatment. It has not given any information to physicians on the diet, enzyme treatment, strengthening the immune system, and organ detoxification. All of these things would help cancer patients survive for more than 5 years. The NCI has pushed four treatments for cancer, chemotherapy, radiation, surgery, and cancer drugs. They have not given information on other treatments necessary for curing cancer or to find alternative treatments for the oncologists.

By 1995, 51 new patented cancer drugs were approved by the FDA to combat cancer. Since that time, there have been over 50 more patented drugs approved. When you equate these new drugs and the 50 billion dollars they have spent, these are the statistics to date.

1. The average cancer success rate with treatment for patients living over five years of longevity was 50 percent in 1950. Today there is an average of a little over 55 percent overall success

80

rate, excluding proton therapy. This may have improved a little over the last 5 years, and with some new drugs, but not significantly.

2. In 1950 one in 25 people over 25 years old, were diagnosed with cancer. Today that figure is one in two for men and one in three for women

In 1950, the dollar amount spent on cancer research was 80 percent less than has been spent in the last 10 years. The question is: Why has the success rate for patients living over 5 years or more, almost the same, or just a little better in the last 70 years, since 1950?

4. Why are the FDA, NCI, and the oncologists working only to cure the symptoms, when they know that there are many other homeopathic and plant-based treatments, plus high voltage pulse instruments that have helped the European and other foreign nations cure from 85 to 90 percent of their cancer patients? In the U.S., cancer diets, and alternative cancer treatments, are usually not communicated to the patient by the oncologists.

5. Why has the FDA and NCI tried to restrict or shut down every metabolic, homeopathic, and plant-based cancer treatment, or not used these great treatments to help them to cure cancer?

6. Why would the FDA and the NCI state that there are side effects to the metabolic treatment, when over 200,000 patients in the U.S., Europe, and other countries, have had the homeopathic metabolic treatment and have been cured of cancer with no side effects?

7. Why did the FDA make pancreatic pig enzymes, which have been proven to help cure cancer, a prescription item, when it is a food, and a very successful cancer cure procedure?

Seventy-seven alternate homeopathic physicians that had been curing many cancer and autism patients, have mysteriously died in the last 5 years? No oncologist has mysteriously died during that time. Is this a coincidence?

Drs. William Kelley, Nicholas Gonzalez, John Baird, Johnathon Wright, Johanna Budwig, and many other alternate physicians have cured thousands of cancer patients. They have not done any harm to over 200,000 patients while curing the majority of them. Their survival rates were far better than the medical establishment's treatment.

There have been thousands of testimonials from patients that have been cured of cancer with alternative treatments.

Another interesting note: Medical oncologists receive a commission from the drug companies for prescribing cancer drugs. Many have a yearly salary upwards of $400.000.00 to $500,000.00. The drugs usually range from $3,000.00 to $15,000.00 per month.

The drug companies have given millions of dollars to the FDA, NCI, lobbyists, and oncologists, for keeping the present form of prescription drug and cancer treatment. It is ironic that some time ago, the FDA named the CEO of Monsanto to be the head of the FDA. Quite a few heads turned there.

Recently, some new methods of using cannabis, combinations of chemo treatments, high voltage pulse instruments, and proton beam radiation have been a great help in cancer treatment. I.V. vitamin C and I.V. mistletoe, plus proton radiation have been a great successful addition. pressure on the FDA and NCI may bring on many new modalities in the future. This will be a great and welcome change in curing cancer. Research on cannabis and other plant products may bring some new changes in cancer treatment. It will be a great blessing.

16

Is Fenbendazole the New Cancer Cure?

Joe Tippen's grade IV cancer had metastasized to all parts of his body. After having chemotherapy and radiation with no progress, the oncologist told Joe he had only four months to live. But Joe was not going to give up easily. He had a veterinarian friend who suggested that a dog parasite medicine may help him. The veterinarian may have heard about Hulda Clark's book, which made a strong argument that parasites were the cause of many cancers. The dog parasite medicine that she recommended, was Fenbendazole.

Fenbendazole is approved for parasite elimination in cats and dogs. It is sold under the trade name, "Panacur." Joe was willing to try anything, as long as he knew that parasite medicine would cause him no harm. He decided to use three other supplements along with fenbendazole. They were Vitamin E succinate, bioavailable turmeric (curcumin), and CBD (cannabis oil). He also upgraded his diet, He ate no sugar or sugar products, no omega 6 oils, and very little red meat. He also ate more fresh, raw vegetables, and fruits, raw nuts, and berries. Joe took this formula for three months. To his surprise, his grade IV cancer was gone.

That is not the end of the story. Joe's veterinarian found out that she had cancer. She then used Joe's parasite medicine and his three supplements. You can guess the results. In three months, her cancer was also gone.

That is also not the end of the story. After this great news got out, many other cancer victims tried Joe's parasite medicine and supplements. Most of them had very good results. Since that time in 2017, many studies and research have been done on Fenbendazole. In 2018, a research paper explained the action of Fenbendazole. It acts as a microtubule destabilizing agent, which can kill not only the parasites, but It has been found that the medicine, with the three supplements, gets rid of cancer as well.

Researchers have found that Fenbendazole and Levamisole also act as destabilizing agents, and will work to destroy cancer cells. Levamisole is one of the treatment medicines used for colon cancer. A person may need a prescription to get levamisole.

Before I go any further, let me caution you that the medical establishment does not look favorable on this type of treatment. Without a physician's approval, you may have problems, because this is not an FDA approved treatment. You should have a functional or alternative physician's approval to use Joe's parasite medicine. A person also needs to use the other 22+ treatments in this book, as well. They are all necessary to get rid of cancer.

The dosage and procedures used in this treatment: Panacur–C (fenbendazole) is the brand you can get from Amazon.com or other companies. It comes boxed with three, one gram package. Put one package dose in a small glass of juice (apple, orange, etc.). Drink one package (one gram) each day for three days. One gram is the human dosage, not the dog dosage, which is on the package. Then stop for four days (four days with none). Then start again for three days, then stop for four days. Do this method for several weeks. If no results are seen in one and one- half months, you might discontinue it.

The vitamin E that you need is APOP-E. That has two types of tocotrienols. Take this continually from the day you start on the program.

Turmeric comes in many forms. The form Joe used is CurcoClear. You can also get this at Amazon.com, health food stores, or on the computer. This comes in tablet form. Take 2 tabs each day for the length of the treatment.

CBD oil also comes in many ways. The CBD joe used is EvolvEnterage CBD. Take one half dropper full each day.

Similar procedures and treatments were discussed in a well- known book several years ago. Dr. Hulda Clark, in her book, "the Cure for all Cancers," wrote that many parasites cause cancer. The worst of the 120 human parasite varieties are liver flukes. Liver flukes and many other parasites produce acetyl-aldehyde, propyl alcohol, and phospho-tyrosine. The cancer-causing agents are responsible for causing the "hit," which is the beginning of cancer cell division and proliferation. The liver is not able to kill liver flukes. Dr. Clark's website also has a great parasite supplement. It is called "Intestinal Edge."

Parasites cause many problems besides diseases and cancer. They even can get into the blood and brain. For prevention, it is wise to get a parasite cleansing every year. Also, parasite cleansing, like the process Joe and his fellow cancer patients are taking, usually will cause no harm, so the treatment is not as bad on a person's immune system as chemotherapy and radiation, which is the main treatment used by oncologists. With grade IV cancer, Fenbendazole, along with enzymes (solozymes), 2,000 mg. of vitamin C (acerola) and JoAnna Budwig's cottage cheese, flaxseed oil, kefir, and crushed flaxseeds, plus the other treatments, is usually a benign treatment system which could be tried by every preventive cancer and cancer patient. Dr. Budwig's formula separates "sticky" blood. It separates it so cancer patients get more oxygen. Oxygen is the cancer cell's nemesis.

It may be wise to consider Joe Tippen's parasite program. Look up his website on your computer. His program, along with the 22 treatments in chapters 8, 9, 10, and 39 in this book, have an excellent chance to save your life.

17

Insula Peptide: Is it a Wonder Cancer Treatment?

Peptide drugs, formed by a combination of amino acids, are being used as a new approach to curing cancer without affecting normal body cells. More and more, extensive clinical data will confirm that peptides, including insula peptide, is emerging as a peptide-based, safe cancer therapy. Researchers and some clinics in Mexico have been treating breast, and prostate, plus many other types of cancers with great results.

Using it alone is not strong enough to cure cancer, but with small amounts of radiation, chemotherapy, or cytotoxic drugs, or the 22+ treatment program in this book, it has proved to be very successful in curing many types of cancer. Many cancer doctors say it is a revolutionary cancer treatment.

The medical establishment in the U.S. has not recognized insula peptide as a strategy for curing cancer, but many Mexican physicians call it a revolutionary cancer treatment. Many Americans with cancer are now going to Mexico for the insula peptide treatment.

Many patients who had chemotherapy and radiation cancer treatment in the U.S., were given only months to live. With insula peptide treatment in Mexico, they are still alive and cancer-free.

Insula peptide, with the use of small amounts of chemo, and/or radiation, is beginning to be used more and more. Mexican cancer doctors are finding that it does not destroy body cells while doing a great job of destroying cancer cells. Even in some American clinics, doctors are saying it is creating a new wave of cancer treatment.

There are many combinations of peptide related therapies. Peptides can also be utilized in many different ways, in treating other diseases, and cancer. They can be used as drugs, tumor-targeting agents, treating typhoid fever, malaria, rheumatic fever, and many other diseases.

Research from many hospital and colleges have shown that people with lung cancer, uterine cancer, bone cancer, sarcoma, lymphoma, and pancreatic cancer, have all shown good cancer destroying abilities using peptides with other cancer treatments. They have been able to reduce chemotherapy and radiation up to 80 percent, using the peptide treatment. This is a great discovery as chemotherapy and radiation treatment used by American oncologists, destroy both the cancer cells and good body cells. Insula peptide therapy also does not weaken the immune system, which is a big factor in cancer treatment.

More and more information is being accrued about chemotherapy and the destruction of the immune system. Research shows chemotherapy and radiation destroy the good microbiome, weakens the immune system, plus increase the bad bacteria, parasites, and candida. This is a big, negative factor in the present cancer treatments. When having radiation and chemotherapy treatment, many times the immune system is destroyed to the point that many cancer patients die of pneumonia and other immune-related diseases. That is what happened to my brother, Wally.

Also, radiation and chemotherapy usually kill regular cancer cells, but not all the cancer stem cells. It knocks the stem cells down, but they regroup and return in one or two years, to flare up in the same area, or even metastasize to other cancer metabolism areas.

Patients being treated with insula peptide do not lose their hair, which is a plus in cancer treatment. It also starves the cancer cells of glucose, which is the main source of cancer food.

According to research by the National Cancer Institute, they have been developing peptide-based antigens to induce cancer immunity. When they used insula peptide and other peptides with chemotherapy, it showed remarkable improvement that destroys many more cancer cells than with chemotherapy alone.

Other researchers in the U.S. are now doing extensive cancer research with peptides and immunization. It is an excellent angiogenic agent that is being tested with vaccines, cytotoxic drugs, tumor-associated antigens, radioisotopes, and chemotherapy drugs.

They are working hard to produce a vaccine with different peptides and related products. They believe the method of creating cancer vaccines will derive from tumor-associated antigens. This is very promising, and may very well be the development of a successful cancer cure.

The sad part is, that for now, the FDA, the drug companies, plus the United States medical establishment, do not recognize peptide therapy as a viable cancer treatment. They have a lock on their four treatment systems for cancer and are stubbornly holding onto their cancer treatment modalities. That is why hundreds of patients are going to Mexico to have insula peptides.

18

The Longevity Codes

Part 1

When I first started to assemble the Longevity codes two years ago, I thought it would be a fairly simple task. The more I researched it, the more I realized there was a lot more involved than in my original thoughts.

How many people are interested in longevity? What is your longevity goal? 80 years, 90 years, 100 years, or longer?

Secondly, can I reach all ages from 13 to 90 years? Thirteen year- old children may be able to use this information just as much or more than adults. It may be wise to teach your children about their diet and how it can affect their health and longevity. It should be taught in every junior high and high school.

Thirdly, would you want to place the information on your wall, or someplace where it was available when you or your family wanted it? Parents should not only teach their children about their diet, but understand health, and living a healthier, more energetic, vital, longer living life. It is also good to realize that diet knowledge, energy, motivation, brain function, and purpose in life is partially governed by what you and what your family eats. It is also true that your diet determines how you think, the health of your brain, body health, your energy, vitality, and how long you may live.

Fourth, not only should parents have the discipline to choose the right foods, but to teach their children discipline, so they can choose the right decisions, goals, vocations, and foods for them to live a long, healthy energy-filled life.

When I was a boy scout, the boy scout law inspired me as to my purpose, goals, and discipline throughout my life. Even now, I think of them often. They are: to be trustworthy, loyal, helpful, friendly, courteous, kind, obedient, cheerful, thrifty, brave, clean, and reverent. They are excellent goals for any person to adapt and live by. Although eating a good diet is not included, it is the main force that can direct the boy scout motto.

When it comes to a person's diet, goals and discipline may not be included in the longevity codes, but it is needed if a person wants to happy, stay healthy, have a great quality of life, create and use goals, plus live to be 100 or more years.

Lack of knowledge and discipline is the reason people detour from a great, healthy, disease-free diet, and living a longer life. They stray into poor food buying decisions and poor health eating decisions. This leads to a poor diet, disease, and maybe a shortening of life. Discipline at the grocery store, and in your diet will, in many cases determine your longevity. Don't let the tasty foods in the grocery store lure you into thinking sweet things and taste are better than health and longevity. Impulse buying and unhealthy foods will do just that.

Select your diet goals and stick by your decisions as to the healthy foods that you feed your body. When it concerns your diet, you and your family need to read, use the computer, learn new things about foods, diseases, and the world around you. Also, it is wise to keep up with innovations, technology, nutrition, and health updates. By following the information on the following longevity codes # 1 and # 2, you will be able to achieve the goal of living a long life, hopefully for 100 years or more. Your diet goals are as important as your personal and business goals, purpose, thoughts, body health, and enjoyment throughout life. Your health is dependent upon what you eat and drink.

The longevity codes will help you do that.

18

The Longevity Codes

Part 2

*Diet, Food, and Lifestyle Needed to
CREATE Excellent Health, and Long Life*

1. Try to eat 7 to 11 fresh raw vegetables, fruits, berries, nuts, seeds, leaves, and/or bulbs every day. These foods contain many minerals, proteins, vitamins, enzymes, amino acids, and fiber needed for sustained, good health. They enhance your immune system, help prevent disease, produce energy, and generate a healthy, long life. Salads are a great, ionic, electromagnetic energy booster.

2. Take one, to one and one- half tablespoons of Omega 3 polyunsaturated and/or monounsaturated oils every day. These oils should be kept in the refrigerator. Some of these are fish oil, cod liver oil, krill oil, flaxseed oil. Udo's Choice, and/or northern seed oils. These are highly electromagnetic oils that help prevent arthritis, prevent sticky (homocysteine) blood, which is the cause of blood clots, and radical body cell damage.

3. Legumes and squash. Eat these foods often. They provide fiber, calcium, lower blood pressure, lower cholesterol, and are anti-inflammatory.

4. Essential supplements are needed to assist with your mineral and nutrient needs. Some of the most important are: Vitamin C, folic acid, vitamin B2, B3, B6, B12, calcium, magnesium, zinc, iodine, selenium, D3, chromium, turmeric, ginger, folate, and resveratrol. Iodine is deficient in 52 million people in the U.S.

5. Fish and fowl. These foods contain essential oils and proteins. They are packed with vitamins, calcium, trace minerals, and other nutrients. Suggested to be eaten 3-5 times each week.

6. Garlic is a great nutritious food. It is antifungal, lowers blood pressure, helps prevent sticky blood, supports a healthy pancreas, insulin production, and helps stabilize blood sugar. It is more effective than many fungicides. The suggested use is 3-5 raw crushed or chopped cloves each day with food. Now fermented black garlic is available. That is a good option and has no odor issues.

7. Lemons, organic apple cider vinegar, and limes. These are very important in the daily diet. They help maintain a neutral acid/alkaline balance which is necessary for cell wall permeability. It enables the transporting of O2, nutrients, and minerals into body cells while enabling wastes, and CO2 to escape into the blood. Hydrion litmus paper will monitor the blood and urine, which, if normal, should be 6.2 to 6.8 pH. Healthy blood and body cells need to be 7.35 to 7.4. pH. Too much acidity will increase the chances of autoimmune and other diseases. If you have an acidic body, I suggest, pure, raw lemon juice, or diluted apple cider vinegar before going to bed and in the morning. Barley powder is also a great alkaline buffer. Barley powder (in food), is recommended for raising the pH when the body pH gets acidic.

8. Oral Hygiene. Many people do not realize that excessive bad bacteria in the mouth can contribute to high blood pressure, heart disease, candida fungus, and many other diseases in the body. To stay healthy and live a long life, it is urgent that you brush and floss every day. People who lose their teeth and do not get replacements are at risk of not masticating their food and can have stomach and other troubles. Seeing the dentist for regular checkups and maintenance is essential.

9. Eggs. Eggs produce great nutrition. They provide almost everything needed in omega 3 oils, minerals, vitamins, amino acids, calcium, and enzymes. I suggest 3 to 7 weekly. Lightly soft boil, fry, or eat raw (mix and add to other foods).

10. Fermented foods. Very important for health and longevity. Kimchi, miso, sauerkraut, kombucha, cottage cheese, kefir, etc. Just a little bit each day is great, preferably before going to bed.

11. Sleep. Getting enough sleep is very important for your health and longevity. Children and adults need 8 to 9 hours of sleep each night. It stimulates the action of the head bones, which moves the spinal fluid in the brain and spinal cord, cleaning out the wastes. A rebounder is also one of the best exercises for stimulating the spinal fluid, which is essential for all people. These things also increase body energy and thinking.

12. Exercise. Everyone needs exercise 4-7 times a week for 25 minutes to one hour. It is beneficial for all people from 6 to 100. Running, walking. swimming, jogging, rebounding, hill climbing, weight lifting, etc. All of these helps muscle strength and O2. It is excellent for the whole family, plus increases longevity.

13. Relaxation. Most centenarians have relaxing methods which are very good for health. Dancing, yoga, meditation, reading, painting, laughing, etc. are all good ways to stop and enjoy the wonderful world of life. You will live longer too.

14. Social networking: Believe it or not, researchers have found that most people, who live a long life, enjoy other people and social events. Your church, other organizations, picnics, and family gatherings, are all great. All these things help a person to reduce stress, relax, and enjoy life.

15. Raw nuts. Don't forget to eat 2 -3 (of each) raw (not cooked) almonds, walnuts, pecans, pumpkin and sunflower seeds, etc., each day. These contain protein, polyunsaturated oils, vitamins, minerals, antioxidants, etc.

16. Wobenzym-N. One of the greatest supplements you can take. It contains extra enzymes of protease, pepsin, and other enzymes that help the pancreas in digesting excess meat and other foods. (See chapter 39)

17. Pure or distilled water. Water is man's best friend. Helps clean out toxins from your blood and body cells. Suggested: three to five glasses,

daily. Water helps raise the alkalinity Many people say that distilled water is the best. It is not wise to drink water out of plastic bottles.

18. Barley Powder. Barley powder is one of the best alkaline enhancers. It can be used in soups, and other foods, to raise the alkalinity of the body. It also can be gotten as tablets and used to raise the body pH. A person may need several capsules to reach a neutral Optimum pH. Keeping a neutral pH is very important for health and longevity.

Avoid Poor Food and Lifestyles which Create Disease, Poor Health, and SHORTEN One's Life

1. Sugar and sugar products. Sugar is cancer and candida fungus' best friend. Stop or skimp eating highly acidic, non-electromagnetic, (dead) food made from GMO sugar cane and sugar beets. These are involved with many disease states and poor health, invite disease and shortens longevity. For great health minimize or cut out sugar, and sugar-containing products.

2. Saturated non-electromagnetic (dead) oils on the grocery shelf. They have been boiled to prevent the oils from getting rancid. They are involved in HBP. diabetes, heart disease, blood clots, and coagulated cancer blood. It is wise to refrain from fried and deep-fried products, in homes and restaurants.

3. Red meat. Doctors are finding that red meat and omega 6 fats raise body acidity. Eating over four ounces of meat at one time causes protease overload and toxicity. For longevity, eat red meat sparingly or not at all.

4. Processed and refined foods. All refined foods have no food value. The worst processed foods that are harmful, are bread, corn, and flour products. They turn into glucose in your body. Carbohydrates and preservatives are refined acetic disease-producing foods. These foods plus ham, bacon, sausage, wieners, etc., are responsible for autoimmune and other diseases.

5. Soda pop, diet pop, and most fortified drinks. Some physicians say that pop and diet soda are the enemies of health. Yet Coca Cola and Pepsi are two of the most used drinks in the U.S. Most soda pop has

about one tablespoon of sugar. Artificial sugar in diet pop is worse for you. Chronic use will help cause many diseases and reduce longevity.

6. Smoking, Drugs. Most if not all people have heard many reasons concerning the damaging and sometimes fatal use of smoking and drugs. If you want to live a long time, quit them cold turkey.

7. Pen raised beef, pork, chickens, and eggs. Antibiotics, hormones, and sometimes even the cow and horse parts have been added to the cows, horses, and chicken's diet. Even the eggs can contain hormones and antibiotics. I suggest you refrain from eating much beef and pork, but if you do, natural grass-fed organic-raised animals are much cleaner and better for meat and eggs. Bison are also much better meat.

8. GMO foods, corn, soy, sugar beets, canola, etc., All are seriously harmful. Buy organic, if possible.

9. Stress. Doctors are beginning to write more and more about stress, worry, depression, and insomnia. Stress is now being shown as one of the causes of cancer and reduced longevity. If you want to grow old with energy and vitality, reduce your stress, worry, anxiety, depression, and reduced sleep. Drugs may not be the answer. Take measures that will help. Meditation, yoga, and eliminating stress factors are some of the answers. This is a big topic.

10. Concentrated orange juice, fortified juices, fruit smoothies. You see more and more of these on the grocery shelf. They are not beneficial to your health and longevity. Make your juices with raw, fresh fruits in your juicer, blender, or mixer.

11. Hard alcohol. Although George Burns lived for over 100 years, that does not mean that hard alcohol is good for you. Some wines have polyphenols, but mixed drinks should only be used on special occasions.

12. Margarine, Crisco, omega 6 fats. Margarine, Crisco, pam, and most omega six fats, including bacon grease are acidic, non-electromagnetic foods. For health, they should be kept in the grocery store and not the home. Coconut oil, palm oil, and butter are much better for cooking. Most omega 6 fats should be avoided.

13. Hamburgers, DEEP fried chicken, fish, potatoes, and other DEEP fried foods. These non-electromagnetic (dead), oil prepared foods, should be avoided by all people who are health conscious. Excessive consumption not only will cause heart and other diseases but will shorten one's life. I know it is hard to ignore at picnics and special occasions, but you should eat them very sparingly.

14. Pies, cakes, puddings, and sugared desserts. I mentioned before about sugar and sugar products. Sugar, plus omega 6 oils, are the most devastating disease-causing foods. The average consumption of sugar in the U.S. is about 120 lbs. of sugar/ per person per year or about 22 teaspoons per day/ per person. These are acidic, non-electromagnetic, (dead) foods that are very harmful to your health and longevity. 200 years ago, there was very little diabetes. Now, 35 percent of people in the U.S .have diabetes.

15. Preservatives, colorings, artificial sweet products, and other additives. These are non-electromagnetic additives that have no energy or health value. Store-bought, canned foods, sauces, and flavorings have many of these no value additives. You should avoid them. It is wise to can or freeze all food yourself to preserve the good vitamins, minerals, enzymes, and other nutrients.

This is a summary of most things needed to live a long vitality packed life, lasting hopefully, for 100 years. I hope you save these longevity codes and use them wisely. You and your family will be glad you did.

I have not added the use of stem cells and other telomere lengthening methods, being used by the billionaires, and people who pay thousands of dollars to stay young. Telomerase and stem cells add extra years to a person's life, but they are very expensive and are not within the reach of most people. Also, the things I have mentioned in this chapter, are everyday things that are the true, basic, necessary foods, supplements, and minerals needed to live a long life. They should be the fundamentals that are very necessary to stay energetic, increase vitality, stay healthy, disease-free, and live a long life. If you can afford stem cells, telomere lengthening, telomerase, and other methods of extending life, then it may be helpful. More and more life-extending methods are being introduced.

19

The Human Body, A Parasite's Paradise

Parasite issues are huge. Over 60 percent of Americans host one or more parasites in their bodies. There are over 120 species of parasites that invade the human body. The more prevalent ones are liver flukes, roundworms, pinworms, flatworms, tapeworms, dog heartworms, candida Albicans, amoeba, hookworms, and Ascaris (brain and lung parasites).

All of these little creatures love humans. Many different species live in the small intestines, liver, uterus, kidneys, lungs, under the skin, and even in the brain. Because very few live in the large intestine, stool tests do not always detect many species. Also, laboratory parasite tests do not pick up a lot of parasites because.

1. The specimens may not be tested for several hours. During that time, many eggs and larvae are not distinguishable.

2. Parasites in the liver, kidneys, uterus, brain, and small intestine are very hard to test.

3. Some parasites have three to four-week parasite cycles. Some cycles are not in the visible window when testing.

4. Most elimination techniques use toxic patented drugs. Most drugs will only destroy certain strains. Also, many physicians do not keep giving the drugs throughout the life cycle of the parasites and beyond. Recurrence can occur over as much as a year for some species. Liver flukes have 6 life cycles that last over 4 weeks, and after elimination, they need to be checked for recurrence.

5. Herb treatment will kill over 100 strains at one time, and some other methods are much more effective in eliminating the many strains of parasites.

6. When parasites are in the small intestine for a long time, the toxins mix with bad bacteria. This toxin mix can lead to erosions and leaks in the walls of the intestines (leaky gut) releasing the parasite's larvae and eggs into the blood. They are then free to go all over the body.

7. Dr. Jay Davidson, a preventive physician, states that parasites produce many symptoms in the body. Some of these are irritable bowel syndrome, colitis. sleep issues, diarrhea, brain fog, depression, anxiety, acne, and stomach issues. Dr. Davidson states that many foods and supplements suppress and kill parasites. One of these is garlic. Most parasites do not live with garlic. 3 to 5 raw fresh crushed garlic cloves a day in food are great to stop parasites. Other foods that help kill parasites are beets, vitamin C, fermented foods, raw fresh vegetables, wormwood capsules, tincture of black walnut, berberine, oregano oil, fenbendazole, caprylic acid, coconut oil, ornithine, enzymes (Wobenzym-N), and, crushed cloves. One great thing about many vegetables and other fiber is that it keeps a steady progression of fiber moving through your intestines. It helps in eliminating twice daily, which helps prevent parasites.

8. There are several flaws in the methods that doctors use to test and eliminate parasites. Parasites have life cycles, some that involve three to four weeks. Liver flukes have six life cycles, over four weeks. A problem is that parasite eggs will perish and shrivel up when exposed to air for a short time, and if a stool test is delayed, they cannot be detected. Many laboratory techniques do not perform the tests for several hours or days. The eggs and larvae are then very hard or impossible to see in the microscope. Another problem is that parasites in the small intestine, liver, brain, and skin are usually not tested. Some parasites have very small eggs, and larvae, so some tests do not even find them.

9. Most physicians use patented drugs instead of herbal formulas. This is a disadvantage because most drugs are zeroed in on certain parasites, and do not reach a broad spectrum of them.

10. When parasites are not eliminated in the intestines for a long period, the parasite toxins mix with the bad bacteria. This mix is very detrimental to the thin walls of the small intestine. A leaky gut (holes in the lining) will enable the eggs and larvae to get into the blood. From there the eggs and larvae can go to the liver, body cells, kidneys, uterus, and even the brain. The toxins can also disturb the chemicals in the cell mitochondria and cause a "cancer" hit.

11. Hulda Clark, in her great book, "The Cure for all Cancers," claims that most cancers are caused by propyl alcohol and liver flukes. She claims that when liver flukes can establish residence in the liver, kidneys, or uterus, it can cause cancer. Isopropyl alcohol, loved by parasites, comes in some forms of hair spray, shampoo, body lotions, shaving creams, and rubbing alcohol. It is wise to try to eliminate the use of propyl and isopropyl alcohol.

12. Dr. Clark states that her herbal formula will kill 100 different parasites with one formula. She is adamant that when getting rid of liver flukes, you will get rid of cancer. She treated one hundred cases of cancer, on people that she found had liver flukes. When she eliminated the liver flukes, the cancer was also eliminated. I will not vouch for that, (it's in her book) but it is a very strong argument that getting rid of parasites (especially liver flukes) is crucial in preventing cancer, and in cancer treatment. She uses the separated formula for one month, twice a year, and then advocates a maintenance program in between. The formula kills all of the stages that parasites go through. She says that a maintenance program should be used for at least a year, just to make sure that the parasites are eliminated, then repeated every two years, or if symptoms reappear. Hulda uses four main ingredients to kill parasites, plus some minor ingredients. The five main ingredients are wormwood capsules, crushed cloves, to kill the larvae and eggs, caprylic acid (as found in coconut oil), tincture of black walnut, and intestinal edge.

13. Other vitamins and herbs that help these ingredients are 1. Red clover blossoms. They contain an inhibitor of ortho-phosphate-tyrosine, (aflatoxin) which is the ingredient in propyl alcohol, body lotions, and shampoos. You can usually buy the red clover blossoms capsules at

the health food store. 2. Garlic or garlic tablets. Four to five fresh raw crushed garlic cloves, every day in your food is a great help in getting rid of parasites. It is a great preventer of both, cancer and parasites. 3. Vitamin C, 1000 t0 2000 mg daily, which is great for many things besides parasite elimination.

14. With parasites, Vitamin C seems to quickly help the liver with aflatoxin detoxification. Aflatoxin B is present in all people with liver flukes and most cancer patients where propyl alcohol (from lotions and shampoos) accumulates. Dr. Clark recommends that cancer and parasite patients take Vitamin C at every meal, or take the time-release tablets. 4. Wheatgrass juice. 5. Seven to eleven raw, fresh vegetables and fruits daily. The vegetables not only provide the vitamins, amino acids, enzymes, and other nutrients you need but also contain the fiber that will move your stool daily, clean your intestines and smooth out your diverticulum (folds) in your small intestine. Cleaning out the gut daily (stool elimination), makes it difficult for many different species of parasites to invade or stay in your body. 6. Enzymes. I have mentioned enzymes many times in my book. Wobenzym-N purchased online, is not only is a great cancer-preventive supplement but also helps in parasite eradication. Turmeric also is a great supplement. It not only helps provide NO2 and oxygen but helps get rid of parasites.

15. One other great parasite supplement is fenbendazole. Not only is it a great parasite cleanser, but works to get rid of cancer.

A person can read all about fenbendazole in Chapter 16.

20

The Hidden Enemy that Lurks in Your Brain

Everyone should be very worried about the epidemic of cognitive decline and brain disorders in the United States. Dementia and Alzheimer's disease seems to be cropping up everywhere. Smack dab in the middle of this cognitive decline is the lack of nutritional knowledge, clever refined food, and processed food marketing plus lack of buyer restraint.

By now you know the evils of SUGAR. The average American consumes about 22 teaspoons a day or about 120 lbs. of SUGAR per year. It is by far the biggest threat to your health and the health of your brain. Diabetes and heart disease are also connected to this one disease factor, called body cell "INSULIN RESISTANCE"

Researchers at Tel Aviv University in Montreal checked 500 patients and their diet for over 20 years. They found that the people who consumed the most sugar products had the highest level of "insulin resistance." As they consumed more sugar, their cognitive abilities DECLINED with relation to the sugar products they consumed.

Tests at the University of Washington even suggested that Alzheimer's disease is becoming known as "Type Three Diabetes." University of Washington researchers demonstrated that when levels of glucose in the blood climb it increases the AMYLOID PLAQUE in the brain. Insulin dysfunction and amyloid plaque disrupt the memory by inflammation, and radical cell damage, changing the DNA plus changing the chemical makeup of the neurons, and synapse. The chemical, acetylcholine, which is essential in the chemical synapse connection process, is altered. As chemical reactions change, the result is shorting out the electrical connection between the neurons and the axons, plus atrophy of some brain cells, cell death, plus the related metabolic and cell breakdown of systems in the brain. This process also starves the neurons of energy and leads to cognitive decline, memory loss, and Alzheimer's disease.

To summarize, a poor diet, including sugar, too much glucose, insulin resistance, restriction of body cell insulin, and production of amyloid plaque changes the neuron energy and chemical balance. People need to realize that most bread and flour products change to glucose in your digestive tract. Your poor pancreas needs a larger insulin factory to keep up with the glucose and "glycation" products produced from sugar, flour products, and bread. Remember that sugar and flour products are also the shadow dancers in the causes of heart disease and cancer. High sugar consumption is the cause of high "sugar spikes" in the blood. High sugar spikes are the cause of "insulin resistance." Most memory loss can be contributed to high sugar spikes and glucose from most bread and flour products. If you, your relatives, or friends are starting to get memory loss, the first step in having a healthy brain is to change the diet. Here are some suggestions to stop "insulin resistance" and amyloid plaque buildup.

1. Reduce drastically all sugar, bread and flour products, omega 6 oils, and trans fats. Cut down on red meats, bacon, sausage, and ham.

2. Eat a raw plant-based diet to strengthen and fortify your brain. That includes raw nuts, vegetables, fruits, berries, leaves, grains, seeds, legumes, lemons, and polyunsaturated oils. For lunch, raw fresh cut-up veggies, homemade soups, and salads are great.

3. Try to stop or reduce red meat, sausage, cured meats, and deep-fried foods.

4. As a person gets older, supplements are needed to bolster up the immune system and brain. Some, but not all of these supplements are Vitamin C, B6, B12, folic acid, D3, Calcium, magnesium, turmeric, L-arginine, and iodine.

5. Exercise helps the circulation of the brain. A person should try to get at least 20 minutes of exercise every 3 to 7 days. If you can have exercise

every day for about 20 to 30 minutes that is even better. The rebounder is a great thing for brain health because it helps move the spinal fluid, which cleans the brain.

6. Brain exercises are also a great way to strengthen your memory. Crossword puzzles, card games, mathematics, retaining names, and reading all help to retain your memory and cognitive function.

7. Television and continued long term texting or cell phone use is not helping your memory and reduces cognitive function.

8. Getting enough sleep also is very important for enhancing your memory and brain function. At night your lymphatic system carries the wastes and toxins from your brain and spinal system. At least 7 or 8 hours of sleep greatly enhances the work of the lymphatic system. It also increases neural activity.

There you have it, a way to stop dementia and mental decline and stay healthy with a great immune system. Following the suggestions above will also keep your brain functions, memory, and cognitive function sharp, and well into your old age. A healthy diet, body, and brain exercise, plus reducing sugar products and carbs are the key to a healthy, alert, and cognitive thinking brain.

21

A Cancerous Endopathic Destruction Epidemic is Invading America

The United States is very sick. The five tentacles of endopathic disease are now affecting every citizen in the United States.

This cancerous epidemic is reaching the heart and brain of every American. It involves five deep-rooted invasive tentacles, greed, money, power, control, and deception. It has metastasized into the government, laws, medicine, religion, and even the fabric of many families, friends, and neighbors. Only intensive surgical measures, with truth, knowledge, logic, honesty, love, faith in God, and the constitution, plus changes in many bad judges and bad laws will keep our freedom, and the current constitutional government free from endopathic disaster, and maybe demise.

The split personality of our two parties in our government is causing a rift greater than the San Andreas fault. The sick impeachment and hate epidemic is tearing our nation's progress to a standstill, and it looks like it will continue for many more years. The stress of fake news, lies, treason, and corruption is reaching epic proportions. The sick media, lies, power grabs, drug cartels, prevalent congressmen's greed, and fraudulent control is a cancerous disease that may never be cured.

The winner of this terrible sickness maybe is China and Russia. They are forging ahead with their education, economies, technology theft, monetary preparations, land grabs and power plays that will possibly overtake America in the next five years. Even worse, they may be a threat to world peace.

Inside the United States, powerful institutions are in the "influence business," whose job it is to influence, lie, manipulate and change the beliefs, values, and actions of many of our students and citizens. This is becoming a serious problem. Powerful billionaires, with their socialist, and "one-world government" philosophy, plus population control, are producing a very sick army of followers.

George Soros has now injected over 200 million dollars this year into his 20+ different cancer-causing, and manipulating organizations, to perpetuate the metastasizing socialism, and one-world government. His goals are to control our government and try to change the laws of our great land from the constitution and amendments of the constitutional government to a socialist, non-constitutional, world government. Soros's "Open Society Institute," has total assets of 1.9 billion dollars. He has a big influence in higher education and is funding many book companies that publish books for colleges and some high schools.

Since the 1970s, education in the United States has seen a systemic reduction of critical thinking. The high school and college teaching systems are way down on the list of educational learning, compared with other nations of the world. One of the most serious problems in many schools is that the physics, math, chemistry, technology, 5 G, GPS technology, artificial intelligence, blockchain technology, nutrition, and science classes have been reduced, from required or essential classes to a less important requirement. Social studies, computer science, government, law, general subjects, LBGT, and sex classes seem to be the norm. In other nations, including China, Russia, and many far eastern countries, essential classes are now required because those subjects are the important basis for knowledge and discoveries. New knowledge and discoveries increase economies and create wealth, which the United States and many nations have discovered. When I was in South Korea, the children were going to school at 7:00 in the morning. They were coming home after 4:00 in the afternoon.

Much of the medicine in our nation has also been a sick deceiving business since John D. Rockefeller started the petrochemical form of medical treatment over 100 years ago. The drug companies, FDA, and Oncologists have a lock on drugs and cancer treatment. This is costing patients and insurance companies billions of dollars. Preventive nutrition, alternate medicine, and homeopathic medicine have been brushed aside by the medical establishment, government, and the FDA. It is also restricting the research on new alternative, and homeopathic treatments.

Our government should be making changes in our drug and medical system instead of waging the sick impeachment war. The impeachment and get rid of the president at any cost, is costing the U.S. many productive years, billions of taxpayer dollars, and most importantly, good, honest, well-needed laws. We need changes in the power, greed, and control motives of subversive elements in our government. This would help every citizen of the U.S.

The attempted political power, greed, control, and money laundering, plus the impeachment process, fragments the governments into opposite partisan divisions. These endopathic infectious actions are tearing America apart. The divisions of the two parties create a situation where our representatives may not co-operate together during the many years ahead. This is a sick syndrome that detours and fragments the business of the senate and house of representatives. Also, the presidential races are now a multibillion-dollar enterprise. Wouldn't it be wonderful if that money was used to help the sick and poor families in the U.S.? The nation's progress, the citizens, and the taxpayers are the losers?

One of the most debilitating acts and disease states in America is the attack on religion. Religious freedom is under assault like never before. Leftism is growing to a point that many judges have completely ignored or have even changed religious laws. Much of this is the result of an executive order (law) that Barak Obama signed which allows abortions and LGBT people to invade our religious system.

New York made three laws in 2019 that takes a strong stand against religious freedom. Recently, a leftist federal judge struck down the pro-life laws in New York, implemented by President Trump. Trump was protecting the free exercise of religion, health care, and people's rights. Medical doctors and nurses are being forced to kill unborn babies in abortions. New York has violated the most basic protection concerning people's rights and exercise of religion. Very, very bad!

Obama made another law that ends the ability of churches, schools, hospitals, and religious businesses to employ Christians and people who share the same beliefs about religion, sexuality, family planning, and abortions. It is now a law in New York, that churches, schools, hospitals, and religious groups have to hire LGBT people to work in their institutions. This is a cancerous, sick, infectious, debilitating, and degrading law. President Trump is doing everything he can to abort this law, and curb the abortion clinics which are in many states. These non-christian acts show how much the culture of many Americans has been degraded in recent years.

Another religious disgrace in many states is allowing the use of Sharia law and medicine in Muslim communities. Muslim sex operations on young girls should never be allowed in the United States. Unless Sharia law is curbed, these acts and other ignored Muslim breakdowns in our laws will spell disaster.

Endopathic destruction reaches out to all areas of our nation. Medicine, government, the media, and religion. Many people are targets of this disease. We must reach out to our senators and congressmen. It is a better thing to let our friends, neighbors, and relatives understand what is happening, with the religious destruction, greed, lies, power, control, and subversive division of our government. If more people would use their email addresses to let congressmen, senators, friends, and relatives know of these atrocities, then everyone would be better off.

There is a whole lot to be grateful for. We still have the greatest country, the greatest constitution, constitutional amendments, many great judges, and the best laws in the world. The constitution was written by Christians and has been the law bible for 244 years. No other country in history has had a sovereign government that has lasted for that long. The majority of people are smart and resilient. As long as we understand the problems, we can help remedy them. Praise God for all the wonderful, honest, hardworking Americans, government employees, and Christian loving people in our nation.

22

Cancer, the Disease of Sugar, Carbohydrates, and Oxygen Deprivation

Cancer is a dreaded disease. Now it strikes one out of every two men and one out of every three women in their lifetime. Why is cancer so deadly? It is because it is so hard to detect, hard to keep from spreading and destroy. Most of the time, cancer cells have been in the body thirty-six months before it is detected.

Just before World War II, Hitler was planning to eradicate as many Jewish people as possible. He also was planning and building a war machine in which he could conquer all of Europe. Hitler had many serious things to plan and worry about. He also had a weird obsession that he would get cancer. His mother had died from cancer and he had a polyp removed from his vocal cords.

Although he disliked Jewish people, he knew one Jewish doctor who he thought was a brilliant scientist, and who could find the cure for cancer. His name was Dr. Otto Warburg. He had been working on the origin and cure for cancer for some time. Because of Dr. Warburg's knowledge about cancer, Hitler knew he could not get rid of Dr. Warburg, even if he was a Jewish doctor.

Dr. Warburg was a biochemist and physiologist. He found the people who had a more alkaline body had more oxygen in their blood than people who ate an acidic diet. He then started working on finding why this was a factor in cancer. He found that a diet ABSENT in raw, fresh vegetables, fruits, berries, melons nuts, leaves, and roots (cationic non-electromagnetic diet) had less oxygen in their blood, He then found that cancer cells started and multiplied in a body that was deficient in body oxygen coupled with acidic body cells, deficiency of neutral or alkaline blood (low acid pH). That was a big discovery because he then found that cancer cells, unlike normal body cells, do not need oxygen to start and multiply. Instead, they used a process of fermentation, called glycation, or glycosylation. With fermentation, cancer cells could multiply without oxygen. This was an enormous discovery.

The body gets its oxygen from the air, supplemental nitric oxide, and from the raw, fresh anionic diet that creates and nourishes the body cells and organs. Dr. Warburg discovered that high body cell and organ acidity, created by acidic non-electromagnetic foods, such as excess sugar, carbohydrates, bad omega 6 vegetable oils, excessive red meats, refined, and processed foods would start to increase the process of fermentation in the body cells. This reduces the oxygen supply. It also changes the chemical makeup of the DNA (diribonucleic acid) and RNA (ribonucleic acid) in the mitochondria (inside of a normal cell) to create a cancer cell "hit." Cancer cells then constrict (shut off) the oxygen and ability of normal cell metabolism around the tumor. Dr. Warburg also found that there was a reduction of the polarity and electromagnetic currents in cancer cells.

This process starts with a cancer cell "hit' and metastasis of cancer. Other scientists later proved that Dr. Warburg was right. That after prolonged oxygen deprivation, in an acidic environment, the body's RNA and DNA, in a body cell, would create changes in the chemical makeup of the mitochondria and create a "switch" that was the beginning of cancer. Their experiments proved that cancer cells will thrive with little or no oxygen. The cancer cells would use fermentation to replicate.

Cancer cells love sugar, carbohydrates, and protein from red meat. In the process, they emit incredible amounts of inflammation, toxins, and dead cells. They also kill the live cells around them. This overloads the pancreas and liver. The pancreas cannot produce enough protease, pancreatin, and pepsin to digest the ingested food, dead body, and cancer cells. The small and large intestines become overloaded with toxins, cell lining coating, dead cells, and waste from the body cells and cancer cells. In turn, the liver cannot detoxify all of these culprits and becomes overloaded. All the EXCESS wastes, toxins, and dead cells GO

BACK into the blood and cause radical cell damage plus they destroy more body cells.

That is why it is so important to use coffee enemas to clean out the large intestine and liver. The pancreas depletes its pancreatin, protease, and pepsin, which is the very thing needed to digest the enormous amounts of dead cells, and ingested protein that is used by cancer and body cells. No oxygen is needed for the cancer cells. Oxygen deprivation comes from a bad diet, which needs to be changed, as fast as possible. Pancreatic enzymes are critical and essential help. The pancreas needs lots of extra enzymes to digest an enormous load of protein used by cancer cells (cancer uses the protein from food and body cells). The body cells around the cancer are destroyed by the cancer cells. Also, pancreatic enzymes are needed to digest food for the normal body cells, detoxification of the liver, and cleaning of dead cells in the blood. This is a very important procedure because if the liver, with the toxins, cannot get all wastes, toxins, debris, and dead cells detoxified. The excess wastes, toxins, debris, and dead cells go back into the blood and all over the body. One of the functions of the massive amounts of enzymes is to destroy the dead cells and cancer cells in the blood. Dead cells and cancer cells in the blood are not good and can weaken the whole body. Any person with cancer should understand that massive enzymes and coffee enemas are very important. The massive pancreatic enzymes are needed to digest the many toxic cells and elements that are also in the blood. (see Chapter 8) A cancer MANAGER is very CRITICAL.

23

40 Million Americans Suffer from Autoimmune Disease

What is autoimmune disease? How does it start and progress in your body? Autoimmune disease is a condition caused by a bad diet. Over 700 million people worldwide are estimated to be affected by this "silent" devastating autoimmune disease. It is a condition where your body is attacking itself, trying to eliminate toxins, bad bacteria, viruses, fungus, and parasites in the blood. It is caused by a bad diet, bad bacteria, toxins, intestinal inflammation, and "leaky gut." It can get confused from the cascade of inflammation and toxins that cause heart disease, diabetes, cancer, and other diseases.

Toxins from a bad diet cause Intestinal inflammation. In turn, the inflammation creates holes in the very thin, one to the two-celled intestinal wall. These holes are called "leaky gut' and allow toxins, bad bacteria, parasites, molds, fungi, and other bad hombres to get into the blood. This cascade of toxins and inflammation cause an abnormal response in the blood and white blood cells. These toxins, bad bacteria, etc. overwhelm the white blood cells. There are not enough white blood cells to get rid of the nasty bacteria, toxins, fungi, molds, and other debris. Instead of destroying this cascade of inflammation, bacteria, viruses, fungus, parasites, etc., the white blood cells are overwhelmed. The toxins, bad bacteria, and other debris are then free to attack your healthy cells, joints, and organs. The function of the immune cells also can get confused and out of balance, producing antibodies that attack your healthy body tissues, joints, cells, and organs. Your body is attacked from two sides.

There are more than 75 autoimmune diseases and conditions. Some of the more common ones are:

1. Arthritis and joint disease.

2. Type 1 diabetes.

3. Psoriasis.

4. Thyroid overproduction and destruction.

5. Inflammatory bowel disease.

6. Crohn's disease.

7. Ulcerative colitis.

8. Asthma.

9. Multiple Sclerosis.

10. High blood pressure.

Physicians usually use medications to treat these 75+ diseases. However, the fundamental cause is your diet. Most of these diseases are related to what you eat.

What should your diet be to prevent these autoimmune diseases? Here are some of the most important foods that counteract this cascade of diseases.

1. Seven to eleven fresh raw veggies, fruits, legumes, nuts, berries, and melons each day. Fiber is very essential.

2. Eat very little bread, carbohydrates, refined and processed foods, and foods with gluten.

3. Cut down or eliminate all sugars, and sugar products.

4. Eat red meat sparingly.

5. Minimize omega 6 oils bought on the grocery shelf, fried, and deep-fried foods.

6. Especially if you are over 40 years, take multiple vitamins, A, B, C, D3, magnesium, zinc, folate, magnesium, and selenium.

7. Eat two teaspoons of fermented foods and probiotics each day.

8. Avoid GMO foods. Buy organic. To summarize, don't forget your raw, fresh veggies, omega three oils, squash, onions, garlic, mushrooms, raw nuts, turnips, ginger, turmeric, and Flaxseeds.

Most people do not realize that their diet and the acidic, non-electro-magnetic foods they eat are the reason for swollen joints and other autoimmune diseases. One of the best treatments for arthritis and swollen joints is a product called wobenzym-N. Wobenzym-N works by getting into the blood and digesting the debris, dead cells, bad bacteria, and parasites. That is why the enzyme formula is a great treatment for arthritis and swollen joints. It is relatively cheap and available on Amazon.com. Wobenzyme-N is also a great prevention treatment for arthritis, cancer, heart disease, diabetes, and all autoimmune diseases. My wife and I take 3 wobenzym-N tablets every day.

24

Linus Pauling and His Great Discoveries

Dr. Pauling was one of the most influential and knowledgeable scientists of all time. Pauling's work, because of his chemical, mathematical, and physics background has touched almost every chemistry student, medical doctor, and ordinary person since his great discoveries on nutrition, chemical bonds, vitamin C, genetic diseases, physical structures of molecules, and double helix in molecular bonding, plus much more.

In a vast number of areas, including physical structures of molecules, nutritional therapy, chemical bonding, genetic diseases, theoretical, and applied medicine, biochemistry, molecular evolution, chemotherapy, cancer treatment, and physics, Dr. Pauling made some very important discoveries. His knowledge and dedication, plus his work ethic led him into a physical and mathematical realm where he understood molecular structures, chemical bonding, anion/cation relationships, and innovative principles related to bond networks, structural geometry, DNA, RNA, the resonance of molecules, and much more. Pauling's knowledge about molecular structures and concepts led him to write a book, still used by many chemistry and medical physicians. In 1939, he published, "The Nature of the Chemical Bond, and the Structure of Molecules and Crystals." It was a classic book and is still used today in many medical schools and universities. His work on chemical bonding and modern structural chemistry won him the Nobel prize in 1954.

In 1948, working on a sudden insight and with a sheet of paper, he discovered that a polypeptide chain, formed from amino acids, would coil into a helix structure he called "the alpha helix." The alpha helix is both a globular and fibrous protein that contributes nutritionally to many advances in nutrition and healing. He would have gotten another Nobel prize for this great discovery, but he was delayed in the U.S. from getting to Britain to present his papers. In the meantime, two other scientists got there ahead of him and later received the Nobel prize for the alpha-helix discovery.

Dr. Joanna Budwig later used his great discovery to create a food combination to "unravel" sticky (homocysteine) blood, found in most cancer patients.

Dr. Pauling's scientific writings involved more than 350 publications, while many of his discoveries help people all over the world lead better, healthier, longer, and more reproductive lives.

His work on Vitamin C was a revelation. The FDA and the drug companies called him a quack at the time. But now we know that he had discovered something revolutionary. It is a fact that in high doses, intravenous vitamin C produces hydrogen peroxide, which is toxic to cancer cells.

The FDA and drug companies tried to dupe the public about Dr. Pauling's discoveries. Today, it is coming out and you can find more at www.aacam.org. If you now have cancer and are having chemotherapy, talk to your oncologist about adding vitamin C, I.V. to your chemo treatment. He most likely will say no.

Several physicians and biochemists have now proven that I.V. vitamin C treatment to be very effective. The following exciting story will show the positive and effective uses of vitamin C.

Although Linus Pauling got two Nobel prizes, one for medicine and the Nobel peace prize, neither was because of his great discoveries about vitamin C. It was not until 1964, ten years after his death, that final verification proved that vitamin C was very helpful for the health of humans, virus diseases, plus help treat cancer, diabetes, and heart disease.

Most animals produce vitamin C. Humans are not able to do so. We have to get vitamin C from the foods they eat, drink, and supplements. The medical establishment fought tooth and nail to curtail Dr. Pauling's claim on vitamin C. The discovery was that vitamin C, intravenous, and in doses larger than 2,000 milligrams, helped slow or eradicate many diseases, including cancer, heart disease, diabetes, and infections. He explained his research and findings in a book called "Vitamin C and the Common Cold."

The medical establishment refuted Pauling's claim. They conducted many trials where they tried to disprove Pauling's work, that using high doses of Vitamin C, I.V. did destroy cancer cells and would treat heart disease. However, their research was flawed and bogus. This is the same scenario that the medical establishment is using to discourage the alternative treatment of cancer. The medical establishment and drug companies are still saying that alternative treatment for cancer patients does not work and the doctors are "quacks." This was not new because the medical establishment discourages anyone from trying to change their drug, chemo, radiation, and surgery.

Recent investigations by Drs. Steve Hickey and Hilary Roberts, have shown some interesting findings that refute the previous medical establishment's investigations. They found that the medical establishment, vitamin C studies, and the National Institute of Health studies were incorrect. The investigative works of Drs. Hickey and Roberts are published in a book called; "Ascorbate, the science of Vitamin C." The book has 475 references. There probably is not any vitamin with so many incredible and effective uses in the world. This master nutrient helps ward off and cure not one but scores of diseases. Vitamin C even crosses the blood-brain barrier to help protect brain cells. It will help prevent dementia plus help stop and reverse depression, nerve cell degeneration, and Alzheimer's disease.

Here are some of the treatments and diseases that this magic nutrient can help:

1. It is the best cold and virus medicine on the planet.

2. It can help treat many chronic diseases such as diabetes, heart disease, and Alzheimer's disease. A 2019 study found that vitamin C reduced HBP in diabetes patients. In most diabetes patients, it cut HBP in half.

3. It can defeat almost any infection.

4. For cancer, using I.V. therapy and a smaller dose of chemotherapy will cure cancer with very little damage to the good body cells and the immune system.

5. If CANCER PATIENTS do not use it for I.V. therapy, they can still help treat cancer by taking 6,000 or more mg. per day(of acerola). Once Vitamin C (acerola) gets inside cancer cells, it converts to hydrogen peroxide, which will kill cancer cells. To prevent cancer, it will be wise to take 1000 or 2,000 mg. per day.

6. It is an adjunct to help treat all chronic diseases.

7. Vitamin C reduces a person's cholesterol and LDL.

8. It helps keep a person's telomeres longer, leading to a longer life.

Dr. Pauling's discoveries are being used all over the world. In Europe, many cancer physicians have been using his I.V. vitamin C cancer treatment and vitamin C supplements for many years. Here in the U.S., it may be wise for the oncologists to discover, test, and use some of these treatments to help our citizens. Maybe that will come about.

25

Obesity, Diabetes, Cancer and 120 Pounds of Sugar

Why is it that people do not understand that fat cells and cancer cells love sugar? Is sugar not able to penetrate the human skull and reach the brain? The average consumption of sugar per person, per year in the United States is 120 lbs. or about 22 teaspoons full per day. Who is eating the 22 teaspoons of sugar each day? Is it you, your relative, neighbor, or friend down the street? I'm going to scold these culprits! I'm taking my belt off and laying it on the counter. They deserve a whooping.

What is happening to all of the 22 teaspoons of sugar people eat per day? The acetic sugar, along with refined food and processed foods, forms toxins in your small intestines. The toxins cause gut inflammation. This inflammation creates small holes in your one-celled small intestinal wall. The creation of these holes is called, "leaky gut." Yes, "leaky gut." This allows bad bacteria, small protein and food molecules, candida fungus, and even parasite larvae to enter your blood. These culprits cause autoimmune diseases, plus other very serious diseases. Some of these are arthritis, joint pain, diabetes, heart diseases, allergies, leukocytosis, intestinal colitis, cancer, and numerous other diseases that will start from toxins, inflammation, and "leaky gut."

Many people do not realize that when a person eats a lot of sugar, it produces a hormone in your small intestine which sends messages to your brain. It is saying, "feed me, feed me." This hormone is called "the Ghrelin factor," or hunger hormone. It is a peptide hormone produced by ghrelinergic cells in the gastrointestinal tract. This hormone activates the central nervous system when a person eats a lot of candy or sugar products. This activation is not good for any person. The intestinal bacteria send a message, crossing the brain barrier, saying "feed me, feed me," we need more sugar! The dopamine neurons in the brain activate the need for more sugar. The people with high sugar consumption feel the need to eat more sugar, much like cocaine addicts feel the need for more cocaine or heroin.

So stop! Stop the excess sugar products, stop using the cooking oils on the grocery shelf, excess red meat, stop the deep-fried foods, including French fries. Also, remember that wheat flour converts to glucose in your body. Sugar and omega 6 oils are the worst culprits, causing high blood pressure, diabetes, and blood clots.

When at the grocery store, do not stop at the candy counter. Pass by the cookie and cake table, skip the potato chips. Pass up the sugared breakfast cereals, soda pop, diet soda, ice cream, mayonnaise, cakes, jams, processed drinks, wheat flour products, refined and processed foods.

Also, the reduction of inflated fat cells and obesity is very important. Thirty-five percent of all the people in the United States are overweight, while that amount of people have diabetes and high blood pressure. Bread, chips, bread products, sugar, and sugar products are big culprits.

So stop! Stop the sugar and you will have a better feeling of self-satisfaction, inner control, happiness, and well-being. You may also be well underway to helping stop HBP, blood clots, obesity, diabetes, cancer, arthritis pain, autoimmune, and other diseases.

Best of all, I will be able to put my belt back on, without having to give that spanking.

26

The Body and Biological Ionization (RBTI)

In earlier chapters, I talked about food and how electromagnetic anions and cations produce healthy molecules and energy. The energy is used by blood, body cells, and organs to maintain a healthy, energetic body.

This chapter is about Dr. Carey Reams and why is his work was so important? Dr. Reams was a physician, chemist, agronomist, and mathematician. He developed a non-invasive working test that shows how much energy the body is producing and the amount of energy the body produces, from the foods that are consumed. His results from the Reams Biological Theory of Ionization test (RBTI), not only shows the energy levels of the body but how the body can compensate with different anionic (electromagnetic) and cationic (non-electromagnetic) foods that change the energy levels.

Dr. Reams said that he was guided by God to devise a mathematical formula to determine a person's health and to help the health of a friend's child based on biochemical and biophysical frequencies of living matter. He called his test "The Reams Biological Theory of Ionization." Many physicians and nutritionists say that it can lead to perfect health and prevention of disease if the test is used properly. RBTI testing is a six-part test using fresh samples of urine and saliva.

Six tests are done on the urine sample while the pH or acid/base balance is tested on the saliva. The 6 tests are:

1. Acid/base balance.

2. Body and organ cell debris.

3. Nitrate nitrogen.

4. Ammonia nitrogen.

5. Urine conductivity

6. Carbohydrate amounts.

Doing the tests does not take a lot of time, but the cumbersome part is that the test takes considerable skill to choose the right foods for the correction of the diet to replace the energy lost. The test, when the energy amounts are found, is a way to prevent disease before it gets from the early symptoms, into a full-blown disease. Consequently, the test can find perfect health, if the tester is skilled enough to figure the right diet for the correction of energy lost. Although Dr. Reams had great success in preventing disease and helped many patients to obtain perfect health. The skill to interpret it is why this wonderful, incredible test is not used in every hospital and clinic today. If you are interested and would like to find a few doctors who perform and teach the Reams test, with the correction diet, you can contact Dr.Bob Pike, http://pikeagri.com or Dr. Alexander Beddoe at http://www.advancedideals.org They are both listed on Google.

How does this relate to a person's energy levels and how they can benefit from this test? The answer lies in the acid/base part of the Reams test. This is the acid/alkaline balance or pH of your saliva and urine. By using a test of body liquids (urine and saliva), you are finding the hydrogen potential or whether your body is acid, alkaline, or neutral. The more acidic or alkaline the body gets, the more of an increase in body toxins, gut inflammation, and free radical cell damage. The pH testing is very simple but will tell you much about whether your diet is producing perfect energy balance or if you are eating foods that are producing acidic, normal, or alkaline blood, body cells, and organs. If your pH readings show you have acidic blood, body cells, and organs, it means you need more alkaline foods to balance your acid/alkaline or acid/base imbalance.

40 to 50 percent of all Americans are over acidic. Checking your saliva and urine pH readings with litmus paper in the morning when you get up, and before brushing your teeth at bedtime, is one of the wisest things you can do for your health. It also helps to check your energy

and health problems before they occur. I have been using the hydrion litmus paper for over 40 years. pH saliva and urine strips are measured from 4.5 to 9. They can be bought on Amazon.com health food stores, and the internet. Be sure to buy the saliva and urine strips that show pH ranges from 4.5 to 9. Also, be sure to test your saliva and urine first thing when you get up in the morning and at night BEFORE you brush your teeth.

The lower ranges of pH strips show yellow which gradually changes to green and purple as the pH gets higher up to 9. This is very important: The perfect range for body energy is 6.4 pH. A range from 6.2 to 6.8 is acceptable and shows that you are eating a diet of high electromagnetic foods. Lower than 6.2 pH ranges show that your blood and body cells are acidic, where cancer cells thrive. That means you are eating too much processed, refined, acetic foods, red meat, omega 6 oils, obtained from the grocery shelf, sugar products, and carbohydrates. You also may not be getting enough water, calcium, magnesium, potassium, omega 3 oils. fermented foods, cottage cheese, quark, or kefir, yogurt, fresh vegetables, fruits, nuts, barley powder, and legumes. Barley powder is a great alkaline booster (see chapter 39). One cancer book that tells how to cure cancer with an alternate program, states that a cancer victim if their saliva and urine are acidic, should take 10 to 15 barley capsules each day until their pH levels out at 6.2 to 6.8. then stay at that pH, unless the pH changes. If it starts to become alkaline, then cut down on the barley tablets. Barley powder is also great to put in soups, and other foods.

The pH readings can also swing to the alkaline side beyond 6.8. That also can lead to constipation and disease, but usually not as severe as the acidic pH side. Cancer cells cannot live in a body pH range of 7.4 or higher. Also, remember that hyperthermia is one of the best cancer treatments. At Dr. Budwig's clinic in Spain, a sauna or hot bath is required every day.

If you are alkaline, to get back to the neutral 6.4 reading, some things you can eat to lower the pH are ground flaxseeds, psyllium husks, fish or northern seed oils, and fiber, plus fresh vegetables, fruits, grapes, blueberries, vitamin C, watermelon, cucumbers, legumes, squash, and water. Staying away from sugar and non-electromagnetic foods is always good for helping raise the pH to normal. Raising the pH in the evening: Cancer patients should not eat breakfast cereal, ice cream or sugar products, red meat, and alcohol. Barley tablets and/or one-half cup of fresh raw squeezed lemon juice before bed and in the morning is great for raising the pH. Don't forget that a teaspoon of soda in a glass of water at night and in the morning will be as effective as lemon juice to raise the pH.

Cottage cheese, soda water, flaxseed, fish or northern seeds oils, barley powder, and/or fresh raw fresh lime juice, all help in getting more alkaline. It may seem strange that an acid, lemon juice, can raise the pH, but lemon juice stimulates the pancreas to produce alkaline enzymes, which raise the body cells, organs, and blood pH.

27

The Acid/Alkaline Balance and
The Ballet of the Minerals

The total cancer treatment cost In the U.S. has reached a staggering 200 billion dollars per year.

Most people in the U.S. are tied to the medical establishment system of health care. When we have a health problem, we see the physician. The physician is the first person we should visit. More often than not, he will find a way to cure one's problem. However, one fault of the medical system is that people get tied to the health care the physician recommends. That presents a big problem. If the physician does not mention that your body needs mending by you, a total health flaw is present. The health care establishment many times is more focused on you relying on them for total health care than they are on helping you making you well.

Dr. Sam Queen has isolated the six subclinical defects that are common in all cancers and chronic diseases. First on Sam's list is a pH imbalance. pH is one of the most important indicators of a subclinical defect. Acidemia is present in almost everyone who has disease and cancer. Sugar, sugar products, and carbohydrates dramatically lower the body's pH, causing acidemia. You should check your urine and saliva pH two times a day with hydrion litmus paper. When these readings are optimum (6.2 to 6.8) Your BLOOD and BODY CELL pH is usually optimum (7.4). In an acidic body, when the pH is lower than 6.2, more hydrogen ions are available to combine with anions and anionic sites on proteins. They displace the calcium ions in the cartilage and bone, plus increase the ionized calcium concentrations. This scenario is always associated with loss of calcium, diseases, and possibly cancer.

In cancer, there is usually a severe lack of alkaline buffers which will usually raise the pH. Increasing the alkaline buffers is very important when the pH of the saliva and urine is below 6.4. Some of the most important buffers are barley powder, lactate from cultured dairy foods, citrate from lemon juice, phosphate from eggs, calcium supplements, soy lecithin, and pumpkin seeds. These things will REDUCE the level of free calcium (responsible for plaque in the blood vessels) but more importantly lower the health risk and help slow or arrest the proliferation of disease and cancer cells. Keeping the optimum urine, saliva, body cell, and blood pH are very important in subduing and arresting most diseases.

The Ballet of the Minerals

The electromagnetic energy in food (potential energy), comes from the minerals in the soil. Unfortunately, our soils today are being depleted of minerals. This makes it harder for us to get the minerals we need naturally, even though we may eat a good diet, with lots of raw, fresh vegetables, fruits, nuts, leaves, bulbs, and berries.

If you have the chance to look at neutral (6.4 pH) blood through a dark field microscope (magnified 15,000 times), you will see hundreds of colloidal particles located in the serum of the blood. These are electromagnetic particles moving feverishly in random motion. It seems like the healthier we are, that more of these particles can be found in the blood serum, and the more they move and dance. If we look at fresh vegetables, fruit, nuts, or berries in the dark field microscope we also see colloidal particles, dancing around like ballet dancers in a Russian ballet. The more minerals that are present in a vegetable or fruit, the more electromagnetic colloidal particles that you can see. We do not know very much about these particles. We do know, however, that EVERY CELL in our bodies has a certain pH, or electromagnetic charge, and resonance, or a certain frequency.

Our ORGANS emit certain electromagnetic frequencies different from each cell. Whole bodies emit an electromagnetic charge with even a little different frequency yet. This is sometimes called our "aura." These electromagnetic frequencies determine our vitality, energy, and health of our immune system.

A very healthy person is one who eats a lot of fresh vegetables, melons, fruits, nuts, some protein, whole grains, supplements and polyunsaturated fish oils, northern raw seed oils, cod liver oil, plus small amounts of omega 6 oils, like coconut oil, palm oil, and butter. They also may eat some carbohydrates but limit them because most carbohydrates turn to sugar in our bodies, through a process of glycosylation. A healthy body does not need sugar. Sugar and most carbohydrates have little, or no colloidal particles.

The colloidal particles in the good macronutrients tell us a measure of the health of our bodies, and the healthier we are the faster the colloidal particles do their random dance.

What measures our electromagnetic machines (cells), our energy, vitality, and immune system? It is the acid/alkaline balance of our cells. This is determined by the blood, saliva, and urine pH. If the pH of our bodies stays within the normal electrical magnetic pH (6.2 to 6.8), our cells open their doors to let in oxygen (O_2), nutrients, and minerals into the cells. They also can let out or release carbon dioxide (CO_2), toxins, and waste from the cells. The ideal pH of 6.4 is a big factor in helping the colloidal particles dance.

To obtain the very low resistance exchange the BLOOD pH should range from 7.38 to 7.42. In a very healthy body, the blood pH should be close to 7.4. The saliva and urine pH should then range from 6.2 to 6.8. These optimum pH values allow an easy exchange of oxygen, carbon dioxide, nutrients, minerals, toxins, and waste, into and out of the cells. When these values are all ideal, the colloidal particles rejoice, and a great ballet takes place. Our body cell walls also rejoice when they can easily let the valuable O_2, minerals, and nutrients into the cell and let the CO_2, toxins, and waste out.

The optimum pH of the blood, body, and cells is critical for maintaining healthy body cells, immune system, brain function, body health, energy, vitality, and cancer resistance. This energy and vitality occur from the food a person eats. If the food is highly acidic, then toxins accumulate in the small intestine. Inflammation and "leaky gut" let these bad toxins, bad bacteria, even parasites into the blood. The low blood pH causes the body cell walls to cringe and suffer. When these pH (electromagnetic energy) values change from normal to a higher or LOWER pH then the doors to the body cells begin to close. The resistance of the body cell walls become greater and can cause resistance in the cell doors. The cells can no longer exchange freely the things vital for cell health. When that occurs, a cell and organ traffic jam transfer can occur. Toxins, CO_2 and waste have a harder time getting out. Oxygen, nutrients, and minerals have a harder time getting into the cells. The cells get weaker and the body gets weaker. It loses its vitality, energy, resistance, and lowers the immune system function. Oxidative cell changes occur. Bad bacteria, toxins, and inflammation then cause a "leaky gut" and let more disease into the blood, causing garbage to get into the body.

Our diets determine the minerals, the pH (frequency) of our cells, and the electromagnetic energy in our cells, organs, and body. The colloidal particles also have a lot to do with our energy, but much research needs to be done in that area. We do know that people who get the proper amount of minerals, including calcium, magnesium, iron, and zinc plus the other 63 minerals needed by the body along with a great diet, supplements, and the optimum pH have maximum amounts of colloidal particles, plus more energy, vitality, and a more healthy immune system function. The body is more resistant to disease and cancer. It is also easier to rid a body of disease and cancer.

The pH balance is ever so important because if we get acidic or alkaline (low or high pH), it affects our cell wall dynamics. This slows or even in severe pH values stops the exchange of nutrients, minerals, and oxygen into the cells, and delays or stops the carbon dioxide, toxins, and waste from getting out. The result because of this resistance of cell wall permeability is that the cells get weaker and get sick. This means that the organs, immune system, and body cells and organs will get weaker and sick. Diseases and cancer creep into the body. The colloidal particles slow down or quit dancing the ballet. When this pH and/or mineral, enzyme, and diet deficiency continues, we get millions of sick cells or the cells may even die. With that change, many diseases begin.

When you look through the dark field microscope at the blood from these people with mineral deficiencies, the urine and saliva pH are out of optimum range. A person can see red blood cells that are clumped together, containing plaque, uric acid crystals, poor white blood configuration, and low white blood counts. There is no dance of the colloidal particles. Oxygen is slowed or will stop getting into, or out of the coagulated greenish blood cells. The person feels tired and fatigued. Blood clotting may begin with an abundance of homocysteine in the blood. Strokes, clots, or heart attacks may occur.

In a healthy body with normal pH and mineral content the blood is separated, single, no plaque or uric acid crystals and the white blood cell count is normal. The red blood cells are round and can carry vital O2. Almost all of the blood cells are free and healthy. (See book cover)

To stay healthy and cancer-free you have to have discipline. You have to say no to sugars, pop, chips, deep-fried foods, and excess red meat. You have to limit yourself to certain (dead) foods, tobacco, pot, and alcohol. However, by eating the proper diet of vegetables, fruits, supplements, juices, nuts, oils, vitamins, enzymes, and proteins we can obtain the minerals we need. We then can keep the optimum pH of our blood, saliva, and urine within the excellent ranges. When the saliva and urine are at optimum ranges, then you can visualize that the blood is at optimum pH. You can check these urine and saliva values with hydrion pH paper two times daily. If the values are right on, then the blood values should be on. If the values are off, then you will be able to research with the computer or see your naturopath, and he will help you maintain your optimum blood, saliva, and urine pH. They will give you some foods, minerals, and supplements that raise your pH. Reading the foods, minerals, and supplements in this book may also be a great help. Barley powder and pure fresh lemon juice are some of the substances needed to raise the pH.

When we keep our pH at optimum ranges and exercise regularly, we have fewer colds, flu, sickness, autoimmune diseases, degenerative diseases, and cancer. Every person has the opportunity to keep an optimum pH. But we need to be vigilant and not abuse our bodies by eating too much sugar, many carbohydrates, deep-fried foods, alcohol, omega 6 fatty acids, oils from the grocery shelf, or excess red meat. We also need to exercise routinely to obtain better oxygen utilization. If we follow this protocol we will have a great pH range and immune system.

Now you know how to keep your blood dancing the ballet of the colloidal particles. If we keep them sprinting in random motion, our blood, our cells, our immune system, our organs and the rest of our body will stay healthy. If we abuse our diet and let our cells, blood, immune system, organs, and body get out of pH balance, disease creeps in and the music for the colloidal particles slows or stops.

We in the United States have been very fortunate to have a great system for testing the blood, organs, and body cell health. Hopefully, in the future, much more information will be available for people to assess blood clotting, diseases, and especially cancer. Hopefully, we will be able to find cancer in our bodies before the 36 months that it grows, before being detected now. In the meantime, we must keep the colloidal particles in our blood dancing the ballet of health and wellness.

28

There is a Major Flaw in the Nutritional Education in America

The Blueprint of Disease and How to Live a Long Life

Having major diseases and dying at an early age is the norm for 30 percent of the people in America. The people we see in the newspaper obituary columns are in their 50s, 60s, 70s, and even younger than 50 in some cases. Yet most of these people have the genes to live to 90 and older. What is wrong with our disease rates, health, and longevity?

There are six major steps to disease and the early death rates which should be taught to every person in the U.S. Nutritional education in the middle schools, high schools, colleges, and including professionals is direly needed. Sick people appear with symptoms, and most are given a prescription. Part of the real cause though may found in their lack of knowledge, in eating the right foods to create a healthy body. If that is the case, there may be a major flaw in the nutritional education, and the diets, of people in America.

When we look at the blueprint of disease, we can narrow it down to FOUR MINOR STEPS. They are definite, precise, and simple. Temptation, poor buying habits, lack of diet knowledge, and cunning selling practices. These override the choices of nutritious foods, a good diet, and eating healthy foods for most people. Cravings many times override a person's good sense.

SIX MAJOR STEPS for smarter eating, better diets, health, and longevity are as follows:

1. REDUCE FOODS that cause disease. A. sugar and sugar products. B. Refined foods. C. Processed foods. D. Red meat.

E. Omega 6 oils on the grocery shelf, especially canola oil. F. deep-fried and fried foods. G. GMO foods.

2. The foregoing foods create INTESTINAL TOXINS, which increases bad bacteria, candida fungus, molds, and parasites in the small intestine.

3. INFLAMMATION: The terrorists mentioned in step one cause inflammation in the intestine and erosion of the one-celled thin wall of the small intestine, causing a crack in the dam (holes in the small intestine).

4. ALIEN INVASION of disease, cascading into the blood, with toxins, tiny food molecules, protein molecules, fungus, parasite eggs, and larvae. The culprits go through the intestinal wall (holes called leaky gut) into the blood, then to body cells, and organs.

5. TOXINS, protein molecules, candida fungus, and other debris, cause chronic autoimmune and other diseases to occur.

6. Creation of CHRONIC DISEASES: A. Heart disease. B. Diabetes. C. Rheumatism. D. Bowel diseases. E. Cancer. F. Allergies and other respiratory diseases. G. Brain disease such as dementia, Alzheimer's disease, M.S., and others. H. Shortening of telomeres and life.

This is the abbreviated sequence of disease and how it affects humans. Every person who is serious about living a quality life of high energy, less disease, more stamina, and a longer life would be wise to learn and follow these steps to begin the journey to better health, longer telomeres, and a better quality of life. To prevent more diseases in America, it would also be wise to contact legislators, educators, and school boards to urge them to include nutritional disease prevention courses. Other countries have a much better preventive health teaching system, preventive medicine program, plus much less disease.

29

The Importance of Oxygen in the Human Body

Usually, all vertebrates need oxygen to survive. People get oxygen from the air, water, food, supplements, and manufactured oxygen. The more oxygen a person gets, the easier it is to stay healthy. Sufficient oxygen in body cells, organs, and brain will increase a person's energy, stamina, immune system, and even the brain.

One of the most important ways to improve oxygen utilization is to get regular exercise. When a person gets twenty to 45 minutes or more of exercise four to seven times a week, it not only increases stamina, energy, health, and memory but increases the lung capacity and health of the bacteria (microbiome) in the small intestine. This strengthens the body cells, immune system, and ability to help increase energy, stamina, and stay healthy.

Cells need oxygen to produce adenosine triphosphate (ATP), a molecular substance needed for many body processes. ATP provides the energy that you need to support your body functions and brain. Because oxygen is so easily oxidized in the body, it is reduced to oxygen ions and hydrogen peroxide. The hydrogen peroxide then helps reduce microorganisms and pathogens. Vitamin C is a factor here, as it has a boosting effect, by enhancing the production of hydrogen peroxide. That is why a person needs vitamin C. The body cells also need oxygen to help eliminate toxins, waste products, burn sugar, and help eliminate fatty acids. Usually, the more exercise and oxygen a person gets, the better the health of the immune system, body cells, organs, and brain. This also depends on a great ionic electromagnetic diet. Oxygen has recently been found to be an important component of the skin. It also increases cell function, promotes healing, and memory function.

Chronic potato couch setting or not getting exercise (couch potatoes), can affect blood oxygen levels. This affects body cell function, respiratory system, circulatory system, and organs. This also affects CO_2 levels in body cells, which is an unhealthy situation. Body cells that are deprived of oxygen are more subject to weakness, disease, and even cancer.

There are many other great ways to get oxygen for a person's health. One recommendation is to take breathing exercises. A great simple routine is to take this simple exercise every day. You can do this exercise in bed just before you get up.

1. Breathe in as deep as you possibly can.

2. Hold your deep breathing breath for 20 seconds, then slowly release.

3. Repeat this procedure 4 to 8 more times. This is a simple, but effective exercise.

Another simple breathing exercise is diaphragmatic breathing. This engages your diaphragm.

1. Sit back or lie on your back. Relax your shoulders.

2. Place one hand on your stomach and one hand on your chest.

3. Inhale (a deep breath) through your nose, then exhale. You should feel your stomach move more than your chest.

4. Repeat this procedure 5 to 10 times.

Hyperbaric oxygen (oxygen under pressure), ozone, and infrared hyperthermia are beginning to be a very useful procedure for oxygen utilization in cancer patients. Cancer cells do not use oxygen to multiply. They use glucose instead. Hydrogen peroxide, produced by vitamin C, and hyperbaric oxygen, help destroy cancer cells. Many cancer physicians and the Budwig cancer clinics are now using hyperbaric oxygen and vitamin C as two of their treatments. The patients are using hyperbaric oxygen once daily.

Many supplements are also a great oxygen health asset. The supplements produce nitric oxide that converts to oxygen in the body. I would recommend taking most, if not all of the following supplements for your health, and also for preventing and curing cancer. Four of the most popular and effective supplements are L-arginine, L-theanine, turmeric, and beet powder. Others that are very important are Ginkgo Biloba, hawthorn berries, D3, and magnesium. Another important group of supplements that not only help separate sticky blood but also are involved in many cancer cellular reactions are; Vitamin C, folate, folic acid, B6, and B12.

Researchers and nutritionists have found that a poor diet and low cell oxygen lead to damage to your body cells. A poor diet will affect the membranes of the body cells by restricting oxygen from getting into the cells and restricts the CO2 from being excreted. A poor diet, intestinal toxins, gut inflammation, and leaky gut also creates radical cell damage in the body cells. This leads to DNA and RNA damage, mitochondrial changes, disease, possibly cancer, and telomere shortening.

A fresh, raw food, ionic, and electromagnetic diet will produce more oxygen, energy, and body health. Exercise helps keep a person healthy, plus helps them live longer.

30

The Serious Connection Between Diabetes, High Blood Pressure, Heart Disease, and Cancer

Many common threads are related to these three diseases, diabetes, heart disease, and cancer. They involve serious conditions involving the diet, blood viscosity, artery, and vein constrictions. All three of these diseases can at times culminate in serious blood clotting conditions.

The treatments for these diseases will vary widely. Many physicians bring blood pressure down with drugs, while some alternative physicians use dietary and supplement treatments, and special blood thinning procedures.

The question is, what are the most important dietary causes involved and related in all three diseases. It seems that the first line of defense should be to stop the bad foods that cause these conditions. The most serious foods involved in the cause of these diseases are sugars and sugar products, omega 6 oils on the grocery shelf, sugar substitutes, excess carbs, preservatives, refined, and processed foods. Also, a person needs to change their diet to raw, live, vegetables, fruits, nuts, berries, garlic, leaves, bulbs, and lightly cooked beans legumes, and squash. Skip the non, electromagnetic cationic diet. Many physicians who treat these diseases, give drugs, and ignore this very important advice?

If you have one of these three diseases or know of someone who does, be sure to have them change their diet. This is the most excellent advice for the treatment of all three of these diseases.

If you have high blood pressure, it is possible to bring your blood pressure down naturally. High blood pressure, diabetes, and cancer provide the link and formation of sticky blood, which causes heart attacks, clots, and strokes.

Bringing your blood pressure down with blood pressure pills may be dangerous. There are four blood pressure drugs that most alternative, homeopathic, and functional physicians say are NOT GOOD for your health. Most western medicine doctors treat high blood pressure with these four drugs.

The first drug is metoprolol Succinate. It is also sold under the name, Toprol XL. This drug is a beta-blocker that will inhibit the adrenaline hormone. It brings blood pressure down but can cause adrenaline problems. Norvasc is the second drug that is commonly used. It is also called Amlodipine, Tekamlo, and Lotrel. It is a channel blocker and has been known to cause swollen ankles, headaches, depression, anxiety, and diarrhea.

Diuril or Chlorothiazide is the third blood pressure drug used by many physicians. It is also called Losartan, and Valsartan. Diuril can cause bad headaches, blurred vision, upset stomach, and seizures. Diuril is a diuretic, or "water pill." It flushes excess water and salt out of your body. That means it will also flush out your electrolytes, which your body needs to maintain your heart rhythm.

Another blood pressure drug, Zestril, Prinivil, or Lisinopril, is an ace inhibitor, which blocks the enzyme which controls your blood vessels, and dilates them. It has also been known to cause a rapid loss of your blood pressure. Other complaints are vomiting, kidney failure, and even heart attacks.

The underlying cause of high blood pressure can be brought down with a dietary solution. For those who are taking these blood pressure pills now, it doesn't mean you have to stop them. With a blood pressure-lowering diet, you can adjust the dosage as your blood pressure drops. If you are taking a high blood pressure medication, You must continue to take it until your blood pressure drops. This is very important, as you do not want your blood pressure to rise.

First, I would like to suggest a food formula that would not only help bring down blood pressure but would help diabetics and prevent cancer as well. It is Dr. JoAnna Budwig's cottage cheese, flaxseed oil, Quark, and crushed flaxseed combination, which helps unravel sticky blood in cancer patients. Heart patients and diabetics need to be aware of sticky blood also, as it causes blood clots, heart attacks, strokes, and clots in the legs and eyes

One procedure that Dr. Budwig's clinic recommends is to put 3 drops of celery seed essential oil under the tongue and hold for 30 seconds, then swallow. Do this 3 times a day and your high blood pressure should be back to normal in a few days. For maintenance take this celery seed essential oil once a day.

Other blood pressure lowering foods: white cheeses, 8 to eleven raw fresh fruits and vegetables daily, raw almonds, pecans, walnuts, butter, crushed raw garlic with food, even juicy farm raised steaks (once in a while), fresh raw lemon juice, fish, fowl, oatmeal, barley powder, and legumes. These combat the three coagulating blood diseases that raise your blood pressure, and cause heart disease, strokes, heart attacks, diabetic clots, and stick blood in cancer patients. (see the cover of the book)

Several supplements can provide more oxygen by dilating blood vessels. They produce nitric oxide, which converts to oxygen in your body. These are L-arginine, Ginkgo Biloba, L-theanine, turmeric, folate, beetroot powder, vitamin C, folic acid, B6, and B!2.

Don't forget the nasty culprits that were mentioned in the first part of this chapter. Sugar, omega 6 vegetable oils, diet pop, preservatives, pastries, and deep-fried in oil, foods. They are nasty culprits.

31

The Importance of Your Intestinal Bacteria (Microbiome)

What you fed your microbiome last night is critically important because your intestinal bacteria are the central headquarters and command center for your body health, mental health, immune system, and even your longevity. If you didn't feed them electromagnetic (anionic) raw fresh and fermented food last night or this morning, you are missing one of the most important segments of your health.

I have mentioned the virtues of fermented foods before, but the importance of these foods is so vital and important, that every health, conscious person should have several varieties in their refrigerator. If your refrigerator is missing these important foods, I suggest that you start with kimchi, sauerkraut, kombucha, plain kefir, cottage cheese, and plain yogurt. All of these important fermented foods and many more, keep your good bacteria ratio in an 80% (good) to 20% (bad) bacteria ratio. This is the ideal intestinal bacteria ratio for good health.

For people who have high blood pressure, want to prevent cancer, or who have cancer, I have mentioned Joanna Budwig's cancer treating formula. Dr. Budwig followed the steps of Dr. Otto Warburg and Dr. Linus Pauling in the discovery of freeing red blood cells to provide more oxygen for cancer and high blood pressure patients. The discovery of the double helix bond molecular reaction which dissolves homocysteine, a blood clotting factor, was one of the most important discoveries in the health of people. Many people with cancer, diabetes, and high blood pressure have sticky blood. Even to prevent cancer, and provide a great ratio of good bacteria to bad bacteria, this is very important for your blood and the intestinal microbiome. Eating this mixture four to seven times each week has numerous advantages.

Fermented foods, probiotics, plus a live food or keto diet, provides an electromagnetic energy boost that can shift the numbers of good bacteria in your gut. They help produce billions of bacteria that detour toxins, inflammation in your gut, and leaky gut.

A very important intestinal percentage of good bacteria (80 percent) to bad bacteria (20 percent) is one of the most important steps to staying healthy. Having eighty-percent or more of good bacteria in your small intestine will enhance your health, help control disease, create better thinking, reduce Alzheimer's disease, help stop depression, help eliminate parasites, help the immune system, and help combat other diseases.

You can buy many fermented foods at the health food store, on the computer, and many grocery stores. There are several forms of miso, tempeh, Limburger cheese, pickles, pickled veggies, asparagus, kombucha, kefir, kimchi, and cottage cheese. You should always buy the plain, no sugar, and nonsweet varieties. If they have probiotics or good intestinal bacteria, that is also great.

You can also make cultured fermented foods. If you have a garden, it is a good way to preserve and store in the refrigerator, these great fermented foods. Cucumbers, carrots, kohlrabi, and asparagus are good foods to use. Look upon the computer to see what ingredient is needed to ferment and culture these vegetables (vinegar, salt, garlic peppers, etc.). Your computer will also have information on the many forms of fermented vegetables that I have not listed today.

You can ferment in pint jars, quart jars, and bigger containers if you prefer. One of the big advantages of these cultured, fermented foods is that they raise your body's alkalinity or pH. Most people have an acidic body. Keeping your ideal pH at 6.2 to 6.8 is very important for your health.

It is good to ferment all foods in glass jars or porcelain crocks. Plastic jars are not a good thing in which to ferment your vegetables.

Your 25+ trillion bacteria will thank you for all of the helpful, healthful electromagnetic, and fermented foods that you give them.

32

Don't Neglect Your PANCREAS

No other body organ except the heart and liver works as hard as the overworked pancreas. The pancreas is about the size of a lemon, but its duties overwhelm all other body functions.

The pancreas is very unique because it is involved with both the digestive (exocrine) system and the endocrine system. It produces protease, which digests protein, amylase, which digests carbohydrates, lipase, which digests fats, plus pancreatin (protein) pepsin (dual) chymotrypsin, trypsin, and other enzymes. The pancreas also produces two very important hormones, insulin, and glucagon. Insulin and glucagon both help regulate blood sugar levels. However, both together can only produce enough hormones to digest about four ounces of sugar (glucose). When a person eats a candy bar or chronic amounts of other sugared desserts over four ounces, the remaining amount goes into the blood and to the liver, causing havoc with a person's blood sugar, possibly leading to diabetes.

Controlling insulin is one of the most important tasks a person can do for their health. Why? Because excess sugar and carbohydrates make the pancreas work overtime, producing more and more insulin.

Here lies the problem. Too much insulin production overwhelms the INSULIN RECEPTORS in the BODY CELLS. This makes the body cells insulin resistant. So instead of the pancreas sending glucose to the body cells to produce energy, which is the job of insulin, the excess glucose circulates in the blood. This creates high blood sugar levels in a person's blood. This is the scenario that leads to diabetes, inflammatory disease, obesity, plus autoimmune diseases.

But much more damage is created. Insulin is also a storage hormone. The increased blood insulin in the blood starts a conversion process of the excess glucose into triglycerides and fat. This is why 35 to 45 percent of Americans have high triglycerides and are overweight (obese).

What are some of the things a person can do to help in controlling insulin secretion and lowering blood sugar? Remember that high insulin production may also increase blood pressure. Several things will be a great help.

1. Reduce and/or try to stop all sugar, sugared foods, carbohydrates, refined foods, and processed foods.

2. Take magnesium and chromium every day. About 80 percent of Americans are magnesium deficient. A magnesium deficiency will help cause elevated insulin and high glucose levels. Also, if a person is over 55, it is wise to take calcium with the magnesium.

3. Take cinnamon. Cinnamon helps regulate blood sugar.

4. Take vanadium. Vanadium helps control fat metabolism.

Taking these four steps will help a person control extra insulin. It will give a person more energy, they will stay healthier, and it will help prevent many other diseases. Don't forget that glucose is usually the cause.

There are also other problems with excess insulin. It steals a person's body of energy, causes fatigue, and drowsiness. It also makes a person vulnerable to many other diseases, including HBP, heart disease, liver disease, inflammatory gut disease, leaky gut, autoimmune disease, sticky blood, and maybe even cancer. So be very nice to your pancreas. It may be the very organ that can save your life or one that can cause you much grief, tiredness, fatigue, and disease.

When the pancreas is not able to produce enough enzymes to break down the food, it can get inflammation of the pancreas. This results in a condition known as Exocrine Pancreatic Insufficiency (EPI). EPI develops when the pancreas does not produce enough enzymes to digest the food that is eaten. This deficiency can cause pain, bloating, and diarrhea. With this condition, extra enzymes are needed to restore normal function and digestion.

Heavy continued alcoholic consumption and/or a high omega 6 fat consumption can cause the development of EPI, cystic fibrosis, inflammation of the pancreas, cirrhosis of the liver, and possibly pancreatic cancer.

Symptoms of pancreatic cancer; You would not be able to feel any lump or nodule in the pancreas, as it is behind the stomach and the upper part of the small intestine. Pancreatic cancer is tough to detect, although new tests are beginning to find cancer, anywhere in the body. Pancreatic cancer can also easily spread to the organs nearby and the body.

People with diabetes can be more prone to get pancreatic cancer. One sign of its presence is weight loss, diabetes, jaundice, or pain in the upper abdomen area. The pain can spread to the upper back. Jaundice will occur in about 50 percent of pancreatic cancer cases. It is caused by a buildup of bilirubin, a compound of bile. Bilirubin is produced by the liver.

I mentioned before about an orthodontist, William Kelley, who developed pancreatic cancer. After having radiation and chemotherapy, to no avail, the oncologist gave up and gave William only two to four months to live. William, who had nutrition training, quickly did more research on alternative treatments of pancreatic cancer. He then cured his pancreatic cancer. After curing his cancer, he went on to treat his friends with cancer. Soon more and more people with diseases and cancer saw him for treatment. He then treated more than 20,000 patients, with a success rate of 85 to 90 percent. One of the first things that he claimed to be the most important, was the massive intake of pancreatic enzymes that he took. His great cancer cure book, Victory over cancer, can be obtained by calling 623 327 1778. It is a great book on curing cancer with noninvasive alternative treatment.

Endocrine Pancreatic insufficiency (EPI) exists in all pancreatic cancer patients. The cancer cells produce, digest, and use so much protein and sugar, that it leaves a huge pancreatic deficiency. The pancreas

142

cannot produce enough pancreatic enzymes to digest the protein from the dead cancer cells, body cells that it destroys, protein eaten by the patient, and body cells around the cancer cells. Massive pancreatic enzymes are needed to make up for the deficiency. That is why it is so important. With cancer, the number one treatment is to use massive amounts of pancreatic enzymes.

If a person is pregnant, breastfeeding, has a blood disorder, or taking a blood thinner, they should check with a physician before entering a daily regime of pancreatic enzymes.

If you have cancer or want to prevent cancer, pancreatic enzymes are needed every day, with other supplements and minerals. There is a very important reason. Since the pancreas can only produce about four ounces of pancreatin and other enzymes, overeating more than four ounces of protein and sugar, sugar substances, and omega 6 fats, leave undigested protein, omega fats, and other food fragments in your blood. This next part is very important. The pancreatin enzymes digest excess food and protein particles in YOUR BLOOD.

There are two very good cancer and preventive cancer pancreatic enzymes, that can be taken for digesting excess substances in the blood, plus preventing cancer. They are solozymes, and wobenzym-N.

Solozymes can be obtained from www.collegehealthstores.com and by calling 817 458-9241. They are sold by John Kelley, the son of Dr. William Kelley, mentioned before, as having pancreatic cancer, given two to four weeks to live, then saving his own life. Dr. Kelley went on to treat over 20,000 disease and cancer patients with an 85 to 90 percent success rate of curing their cancer. For PREVENTING cancer, John Kelley recommends to take 6 to 8 solozyme tablets between meals each day. Wobenzym-N tablets can be obtained over the internet, and at Amazon.com.

The cancer-preventive dosage for wobenzym-N tablets is three to five tablets each day, between meals. They are very reasonable and can be gotten on the internet and/or at Amazon.com.

The facts above show why the pancreas is the Hercules of body organs. Keeping the pancreas happy is by eating healthy foods, plus not over-eating, and especially overeating with a lot of junk food. If you keep the pancreas happy, it will keep you happy, for a long time.

33

Why in the World are People Dying so Young?

The obituaries in our town are showing many people in their 50s, 60s, and even 70s, that are leaving us and this wonderful world way too early. Many of these people are dying from cancer. A short time ago, one of our dear friends died of breast cancer at the young age of 63. This is sad. This is also odd since many longevity physicians and researchers are saying that our bodies have the telomeres that will last until a person reaches 120 years old. But one big problem is, in over 70 years, cancer doctors have not been able to improve their success rates for curing cancer.

There are many stories about the millionaires and billionaires getting stem cell therapy, I.V. bone marrow injections, and other telomere lengthening treatments that will give them many extra years of life. Many of these people realize that they also have to follow a strict regimen of exercising, eating an excellent diet, and keeping a lifestyle that enhances long telomeres and long life. Your telomeres are the tiny "countdown clocks" that are at the end of each DNA strand, inside your body cells. Dr. Al Sears says "short telomeres have been linked to a 300% increased rate of death from heart disease and an 800% higher death rate from infectious diseases."

Most of us are not able to afford the high costs of taking these stem cell life enhancers to extend our lives. And really, are stem cells that sustain the fountain of youth, going to enable everyone to live a disease-free and healthy long life? If we look closely, we would find the reason for diabetes, high blood pressure, heart disease, cancer, and other diseases that are shortening these people's lives. If we understand what causes these diseases, and how to combat them, then every person has the telomeres to live a long life, but it may not be easy in this complex, sad environmental, GMO. refined and processed food world. There is more diabetes, Alzheimer's disease, heart disease, autoimmune diseases, and cancer than ever before. The center for disease control stated that many alternative preventive physicians are finding that the diets of many Americans are prematurely killing them. One hundred twenty lbs. of sugar per year is what the average person in the U.S. eats. This amount cannot stretch the telomeres into a longer length. The tiny pancreas cannot control the insulin from the bad diet and does not have enough enzymes for an excess of protein. They are finding that "ninety percent" of all diseases can be attributed to "TWO' very serious ailments. These ailments change the DNA and RNA in the body cell mitochondria and can cause many diseases, plus cancer. First, an acidic, bad sugar, omega 6 oil, refined and processed food diet, mentioned many times in this book, produce toxins and "INFLAMMATION," in the one-celled walls of the small intestine. These ornery bad bacteria, candida, parasites, other culprits, and toxins then cause "LEAKY GUT." Second, the leaky gut creates holes in the small intestine that allow the nasty toxins, bad bacteria, candida, other parasites, and every other nasty germ to get into the blood. Diabetes, heart disease, autoimmune diseases, and cancer will follow. The telomeres crawl into the corner and start to give up their long length.

But hope is on the horizon. Eliminating stress and worry can be the forerunner to a longer life. Eating a good diet, with mostly raw or lightly cooked foods, polyunsaturated oils, getting good supplements, minerals, eliminating bad omega 6 oils, and sugar, exercising, plus keeping or maintaining a neutral acid/base balance in your body cells and blood, can change the conditions, and let the telomeres come out of the corner. With these changes, people can live a longer life, and many will also prevent cancer with a great lifestyle, and diet modifications.

Dr. Al Sears has made it his life's work to research and teach his patients how to increase the length of their telomeres and live a longer life. He states that the most critical thing is to know is your telomere age. The shorter your telomeres are, the more you are prone to symptoms of old age. He has several biomarkers that test the telomere age and biological age of his patients. He then helps correct their diets and gives them changes in their biomarkers to lengthen their telomeres. His biomarkers include heart and lung power., bone density and strength, memory, artery health, hormones, grip strength, hearing, and range of motion. These are combined with a strict diet with the instructions that are mentioned above.

Dr. Sears also has some suggestions on how to restore your telomeres. One supplement he recommends is MILK THISTLE. It increases telomerase activity threefold. Silymarin, its ingredient, is a very strong antioxidant that stops free radical damage in body cells. Buy the highest concentrations available because the higher concentrations improve absorption and bioavailability.

Another great extract not only inhibits the oxidative stress that causes aging but lengthens the telomeres by as much as 40 percent. It is an extract from the Terminalia Chebula tree. It is also known as haritaki and myrobaian. It has been used for thousands of years to cure a wide variety of diseases, including heart disease, high blood pressure, asthma, and diabetes. In India, it is known as a great medicine. Dr. Sears says it is hard to get, but a person needs to find a website that specializes in Ayurvedic herbs.

I hope these suggestions will help you in your quest for a long, prosperous, healthy, vital, energetic, and long life. If these suggestions will help one person or more, in living a longer life, it will fulfill my mission. Living a longer life is the obligation of each person, and determines the quality of life that they want to lead. It is sometimes hard to maintain the standards and discipline necessary in keeping long telomeres, but in the long term, it is worth it.

34

The Covid-19 Virus Brings out Extreme Nutritional Deficiencies in Senior Citizens

Many people in the U.S. have a relative or friend in a senior citizen's home. The high coronavirus statistics and contagion that has happened, is a concern and worry for everyone. When analyzing the problem, one might find suggestions that may help in finding the reasons for the high mortality rate.

There are some important reasons for the many covid-19 infections and deaths. Many seniors have underlying problems with their health. In Italy, it was found that 97 percent of all infections and covid-19 deaths in retirement and rest homes were in unhealthy individuals with at least one underlying problem, including heart disease, diabetes, high blood pressure, and other ailments. Many of the seniors that were infected the most had more than one underlying health problem. However, the mortality might also be from the senior's diet, deficient supplements, minerals, and most of all, their weak immune systems.

Why would a person's immune system be so weak that being susceptible to diseases would be so high? I have been familiar with that issue after visiting and eating at several retirements and senior citizen's homes.

In many rest and senior citizen's homes, the diets are not immune system important. In many senior citizen's homes, but not all, dieticians do not set up food menus with the main issue of boosting the immune system. Problems may arise from the ability of the residents having trouble with chewing. However, the majority can chew their food well.

Another problem may be that many dieticians feed their seniors what they like to enjoy, and what the majority of people like.

Emphasis should be on diet entries that boost the immune system. These are foods that contain vitamins, minerals, amino acids, and other nutrient foods. Many of these nutrient foods can be raw or lightly cooked vegetables, fruits, nuts, roots, such as beets, radishes, turnips, parsnips, onions, garlic, potatoes, plus cooked whole grains like oatmeal, buckwheat, ryemeal, flaxseeds, chia, and other small grains. Also, fermented foods can add great benefits. I know that salads are usually available for lunch and dinner. That is good. Cottage cheese and fruits are also usually offered for breakfast. That is good. I noticed that apples, bananas, and oranges are available, but many of the other fruits are canned. According to many researchers, about 40 percent of the nutrients are left after canning fruits and vegetables. It may be wise to offer more raw fresh fruits and things like raw grapes, sliced apples, pears, cantaloupe, kiwi, avocado, and mangos, which have great vitamins, minerals, enzymes, and other nutrients. Is the diet the main reason for the low immune systemin senior citizens? It is very important, but probably not the main culprit for the majority of the senior's susceptibility problems. It would also be an advantage to have polyunsaturated oils available for all residents.

My thoughts are that the deficiencies of supplements, vitamins, omega 3 oils, and minerals have left a vulnerable void of the very things that doctors say are needed to combat the covid-19 virus. These important virus-fighting supplements, vitamins, and minerals are Vitamin C, folate, vitamin D3, zinc, calcium, magnesium, CoQ10, B6, and B12. There is one other thing that Canadian Doctors have recommended, tonic water. Tonic water has quinine, the substance that is in some of the drugs used to help cure viruses.

Senior citizens are most deficient in calcium, folate, vitamin C, D3, zinc, and magnesium. Most young people and even adults have greater amounts of these supplements. The seniors that do not get supplements and minerals may also be more vulnerable to the virus.

Magnesium studies from scientific journals have shown that 58 to 68 percent of seniors have a deficiency of magnesium. Magnesium is a

149

very important mineral because it not only is called nature's channel blocker, but also the main mineral that works with calcium. It performs over 300 other chemical reactions in the body. It helps lower the blood pressure, performs insulin regulation, and lowers hypertension.

Vitamin C is very important because magnesium and folate will combine with Vitamin C, and B12, to help the body break down protein, plus helps create new red and white blood cells, needed for immunity. It helps in the formation of DNA, which keeps the body cells healthy. A vitamin C deficiency can be caused when a person does not eat leafy vegetables, needed for vitamin C and folate synthesis. For a senior to help fight covid-19, it is recommended that a person get 2,000 mg. of vitamin C, 400 t0 600 mcg. mg. of folate a day. Zinc, 50 mg, and vitamin D3, 10,000 to 20,000 IU each day.

Folate and vitamin B12 work with B6 to help stop coagulation in the red blood cells. This is needed for senior citizens to create healthier red and white blood cells, and fight covid-19 and other diseases. The folate dosage is 400 to 600 mcg/day. B12 can come as a nasal spray or tablet. The normal adult dosage is 1,000 to 2,000 mcg per day. Selenium helps fight memory loss, plus improves blood flow. For selenium, 400 to 600 mcg tablets will be a daily dosage.

CoQ10 is known as ubiquinone-10. It is a very important supplement that will help generate energy in humans. It is a booster for the heart, liver, and kidneys, plus a great antioxidant. Dosage is 100 to 300 mcg/ twice daily.

Everyone needs iodine. Dr. Brownstein states that 52 million Americans are deficient in iodine. Yet it is available in many forms. It comes in salt, especially sea salt, Himalayan salt, liquid drops, and as a topical liquid. Senior citizens should have seas salt or Himalayan salt at each table.

I have assembled a lot of information on diet, supplements, vitamins, and minerals. What are some of the options for senior citizen's homes in helping in this troubled coronavirus world?

Here are some suggestions:

1. Even though many senior citizens may not eat a lot of fresh, raw vegetables, fruits, nuts, and berries, cut up portions of these fresh items could be available on the menu, and even FEATURED on the menu as very helpful for the person. If they are featured or suggested, maybe more people would eat them.

2. HIGHLIGHT nutrient-rich menu entries, such as cottage cheese, salads, raw, fresh vegetables, fruits, oatmeal mush, and other foods might bring attention to more people.

3. The retirement or senior citizen's home might write a WEEKLY BULLETIN mentioning supplements, minerals, and other essential nutrients with the dosages and instructions, so residents, friends, or relatives would be able to get them for the people.

4. Some Senior citizen's homes and retirement homes do not have exercise rooms and facilities. Exercise is a major health supplement for all older people. It should also be mentioned in a weekly bulletin. Larger homes could have an exercise manager, one to 4 days a week.

5. Another tip is that tonic water has an ingredient, quinine which can help fight viruses. The rest and retirement homes might have tonic water available for the senior citizens.

6. Recently two other great supplements have been found to help senior citizens. They are ashwagandha and horsetail. Ashwagandha has been found to increase white blood cell count by four times. Doctors have found that a normal white blood cell count can rise from 600-700 white blood cells to 2500-2800.

The other supplement is horsetail. It contains chlorophyll and other ingredients, which also helps raise the white blood cell count. Both are also very helpful in combating cancer.

These are just suggestions to help senior citizens stay more healthy, plus combat the covid-19 and other viruses. Maybe the residents might also have some suggestions that would help to combat disease. Staying healthy and combatting disease is important for the senior population.

Dosages of supplements and minerals may vary from one individual to another. Be sure to check with your physician for dosages of the supplements, and minerals. If a senior citizen has relatives or close friends, they may be a very good help in obtaining supplements and minerals.

35

52 Million People are Deficient of Iodine

Dr. David Brownstein, an authority on the thyroid gland, states that 52 percent of Americans are deficient in iodine.

The thyroid gland is a small butterfly-shaped gland that covers the front of a person's trachea, or windpipe. It releases thyroid hormone which controls the growth and metabolism, of all the cells in a person's body.

The pituitary gland controls and releases the thyroid-stimulating hormone (TSH) and signals the thyroid gland to release the hormone amounts needed to control the metabolism of the body cells. Sometimes TSH levels decrease, not signaling the thyroid gland. This can cause hypothyroidism.

Dr. Brownstein, after graduating from medical school, read the book written by Johnathon Wright, MD. This changed his whole life, and the way he started practicing medicine. After reading the book, he started a holistic preventive medicine practice. He wonders why physicians are not trained in holistic medicine, because it helps so many people.

We can thank John D. Rockefeller for that since he started the petro medicine path of practicing patented medicine in 1878. A pill for every ill.

Dr. Brownstein states that every patient in his practice gets a complete nutritional and hormonal evaluation. He uses serum testing of hormones, hair tests, and urine tests, plus TSH levels. Every patient is checked for thyroid antibodies, testosterone, progesterone, estriol, estrogen, D3, B12 levels, magnesium, zinc, copper, and a urinary secretion iodine test. He also checks the diet, dietary history, hormonal balances, and social issues.

Iodine is needed for more than the thyroid. It is needed for the production of every hormone in the body. The thyroid holds only one percent of the body's iodine stores. The skin holds 20 percent, the breasts hold five percent, and the rest is stored throughout the body. Most people do not realize that a person needs iodine every day. It is hard to get hyperthyroidism.

Dr. Brownstein states that people need at least 25 mg. of iodine each day. It also works better with magnesium, zinc, DHEA, and selenium. Low thyroid is also suspected as a cause of cancer.

Signs and symptoms of hypothyroidism:

1. Feeling tired and worn out: Loss of energy, feeling exhausted and sluggish.

2. Gaining weight: when iodine gets low, metabolism gets low, energy gets low, metabolism slows down, and people feel colder. People store calories instead of using calories.

3. Metabolism is decreased: hypothyroidism make a person feel colder, It slows down the body heat

4. Weakness in joints and muscles: Muscle strength decreases

5. Hair loss: Hair loss occurs in some people. Hair follicles are regulated by the thyroid hormone. Low thyroid hormone causes hair follicles to stop regenerating, resulting in hair loss.

6. Dried skin and itching: Dry skin can also be caused by other deficiencies.

7. Feeling down and depressed: People can also have anxiety and depression.

8. Have trouble concentrating: Some people have memory loss, but may not all be from the thyroid.

9. Constipation: Sometimes, but not always the cause.

10. Heavy or irregular periods: It is best to see a gynecologist.

Dr. Brownstein said it is hard to get enough iodine in the tainted food supply. Most people need iodine supplements to get adequate dosages. Women who get pregnant should start iodine and vitamin D supplements when knowing they are pregnant. He also said that iodine helps the immune system fight back against many infectious diseases.

Hashimoto's Hyperthyroidism Disease

Sometimes, an autoimmune condition mistakenly attacks the healthy tissues of the thyroid gland. It causes thyroid gland inflammation. Dr. Hashimoto in Japan was the first person to describe the disease around 1920. In 1957 it was recognized as an autoimmune disease, after testing for hypothyroidism. It was found that the thyroid needs iodine to manufacture thyroid peroxidase (TPO) which is needed to synthesize thyroid hormones.

A thyroid physician, Dr. Kharrazian, states for Hashimoto's disease a person need not take extra iodine supplements, but to get it from the diet. He contends that gluten and dairy are part of the cause of Hashimoto's disease, and supplemental iodine should not be included in the diet. Cutting down on Gluten and dairy are also recommended for many other diseases as well.

Chiropractors and naturopaths treat a lot of Hashimoto's disease patients, with nutrition and lab tests for finding other deficiencies that impair the thyroid gland. These can be tests for factors like the pituitary gland, minerals, estrogen, testosterone, or too much cortisol.

Dr. Brownfield says the best treatment for Hashimoto's disease is thyroxine T4. However, extracts are also available that are derived from the thyroid glands of pigs. My suggestion is to check with a very good preventive medicine physician when having symptoms of Hashimoto's disease.

A person should also remove any immune reactive foods from the diet. Individual tests are needed to check for allergies.

Several foods are rich in iodine. Some of these are:

1. Seaweed; Kombu kelp, dried wakame, miso soup, nori-sushi rolls:

2. Sea cod, bottom fish: They have a wide variety of minerals including iodine.

3. Yogurt, cottage cheese, kefir:

4. Himalayan salt and sea salt:

5. Shrimp and calamari:

6. Tuna, sardines, and omega 3 fats:

7. Eggs: Usually, iodine is added to chicken feed. Many eggs have around 16 percent of daily iodine.

8. Prunes and lima beans: They also have a small amount of iodine.

Are you one of the 52 million people in the U.S. that needs extra iodine? Be sure to take magnesium, selenium, Vitamin C, D3, B12, zinc, copper, and folate. They will also help many other diseases including covid-19, colds, pneumonia, and many other ailments.

36

The Sad Story of Dr. Jeffery Bradstreet

Our story begins with an explanation of a cancer treatment drug. It is used by some physicians and is called GcMAF. GcMAF occurs naturally in our bodies. The scientific definition is Globulin component, macrophage activating factor, or (GcMAF). It is a vitamin D binding regulatory protein, which is present in the immune system. This naturally occurring protein is found in healthy individuals but is lacking in people with a weak immune system, children with a deficiency of vitamin D, or children with autism.

The following statement is very important. "GcMAF therapy has been shown to enhance the immune system function. It possibly can prevent and even reverse CANCER and AUTISM." The FDA has not and evidently will not test this very crucial important cancer treatment protein.

GcMAF is very important for activating white blood cells (macrophages) that digest cancer cells, cellular debris, and other invading disease bacteria and cells when they are not identified as healthy body cells. When GcMAF is absent or weak, the ability for macrophages to work is negated or weakened considerably.

Vitamin D is a very important vitamin needed by pregnant women, infants, and even adults. The most important form is Vitamin D3, recommended for all individuals. The uses of vitamin D are very important. Its essential use is in the development of the brain, brain function, and memory function. It is essential for all developing young babies and children. Besides being essential in brain development, and defend the immune system from chronic disease, it is very important in regulating the GcMAF function. Most physicians prescribe Vitamin D3, therapy for pregnant women, and young babies. Vitamin D3, GcMAF, and vitamin C are all needed for the development of the central nervous system. The following neurobiological processes require all three: neuroprotection, neuro-plasticity, and neurogenesis. Neurogenesis is the process of creating new brain cells.

Vitamin D deficiency disrupts the proper development of the brain and the immune system. This also affects the spinal cord. It is also the major link in the development of autism. Individuals with autism have been found to have disrupted macrophage defenses. Dr. Jeffery Bradstreet discovered that when treating autistic children with GcMAF, it diminishes the autistic syndrome, and increases the macrophage activity.

Nagalase is an enzyme found with an increased risk for lupus, autism, spectrum disorders, infections such as HIV, Aids, and many types of cancer. Nagalase blocks the natural production of GcMAF, and the availability for macrophages to operate, which is needed for stopping cancer proliferation. Dr. Jeffery Bradstreet discovered that children that had nagalase in their blood, had a greater chance of having autism and cancer. Nagalase would shut down the production of GcMAF. This would decrease the effectiveness of Vitamin D and curtail any macrophages from destroying cancer cells. He found that injecting GcMAF restored the GcMAF and macrophages which gobbled up cancer cells. This not only helped the autism patients but also cancer patients, as well. He treated thousands of patients with incredible success. He should have been nominated for the Nobel prize, but a mysterious death curbed not only his work but his incredible treatment.

In 2015, an untimely, unfortunate death shut down Dr. Bradstreet's great work.

Here is the rest of the story.

In June 2015, The FDA raided Dr. Jeffery Bradstreet's office. They took a truckload of his papers. They took all of his patient records, his results of treatment, his research on GcMAF, and his proof that GcMAF was proven to be very effective in the treatment and curing of autism and cancer. Dr. Bradstreet left town and had planned to stay at a hotel near a lake in North Carolina. He feared that he would be facing a long prison term for using a non-prescribed FDA treatment. He knew that GcMAf was not approved by the FDA.

That was when things got much worse. When the room at the hotel was not quite ready, (or was it?) Dr. Bradstreet left the hotel for a short walk. However, the short walk lasted for an eternity. Hours later, Dr. Bradstreet's body was found floating in a nearby river, with a bullet in his chest. Many of his friends say he was not depressed or had any kind of suicidal behavior. Most of his friends stated that he was murdered for his great discovery of GcMAF, as successful cancer and autism treatment. Since 1990, 59 GcMAF positive research papers have been written.

There are also several other stories about 77 alternative cancer physicians who mysteriously died, between 2015 and 2019. Not many people have read about this because the media has been very quiet. During that time, NOT ONE story had been written about any oncologist who had died mysteriously.

If you would like to learn more, please look up the website of Dr. Nicolas Gonzalez. He died mysteriously when he was a healthy, 64- year old alternative cancer physician. Dr. Gonzalez had successfully cured 85 to 90 percent of over 10,000 cancer patients.

37

An Acid/Base Imbalance, Temporal Mandibular Joint Dysfunction and the Blood pH can Create a Vertebral Cartilage Paradox

This chapter is related to the prevention of cancer in an indirect way. It pertains to the acid/alkaline condition of the body cells and the blood. As mentioned before, most cancer tumor cells start in an acidic body (low pH). The way to find out a person's body cell and blood pH is a measurement of the saliva and urine, with hydrion litmus paper. You should check in the morning when you get up, and when going to bed, before you brush your teeth.

When the urine and saliva pH is an optimum 6.4, the BLOOD and BODY CELLS should be an optimum 7.4 pH. A good normal range for the saliva and urine is from 6.2 to 6.8 (6.4 is ideal). If the pH gets lower (more acid) or higher (more alkaline), the body is then subject to many diseases, including autoimmune diseases, plus regular body diseases like heart disease, diabetes, and cancer. A person's diet controls the body cells, organs, and blood pH.

Everyone would be better off if they obtained some hydrion litmus paper to check their saliva and urine twice daily, when getting up in the morning, and BEFORE brushing their teeth at night, before going to bed. This gives them a monitor of how their diet is controlling their acid/alkaline balance (pH).

This is very important because cancer usually starts in an acidic body, why does this occur? Because when the electromagnetic pH and cell resonance gets low, cancer cells and other diseases can begin to thrive. The resonance and pH of cancer cells are lower than normal body cells.

The healthy goal for any person then is to maintain their saliva and urine pH between 6.2 to 6.8 (electromagnetic range). This creates an ideal body cell and blood range of 7.4 pH. A person's diet controls this pH range. It makes sense that when the body cell and blood pH gets low, cancer cells have a better chance to start in a body. To obtain pH paper, see chapter 39.

When the BODY CELLS and BLOOD get below 7.4 (acidic) then several adverse problems begin to occur. The resonance and electromagnetic energy of the body cells get reduced. This creates resistance in the body cell walls which slows down or inhibits oxygen, nutrients, and minerals from getting into the cells and restricts CO_2, wastes, bad viruses, and bacteria from exiting the cells. This creates a chronic, long time exposure to diseases, including cancer.

The energy in a portion of food is dependent on how many minerals, and how much electromagnetic energy the food contains. What are the foods that are some of the best for raising the body cell and blood pH? Water, barley powder, calcium, along with raw, fresh lemon juice, cucumbers, and watermelon are some great alkaline boosters.

My pH has always been lower than the optimum. For years, I have drunk a raw, fresh glass of lemon juice before bedtime, and when I get up in the morning. That, and barley powder has been the best alkaline booster for my condition. Why does raw, fresh lemon juice raise the pH? Because lemon juice is one of the ionic (acid-alkaline) foods that stimulate the pancreas to produce more alkaline enzymes.

One of the most important functions of neutral acid/alkaline balance is controlling body cell functions and the heart rhythm. A constant blood pH of 7.4 is crucial to maintaining heart rhythm. That is where a serious condition can occur which relates to the dental bite, temporal mandibular joint, the neck muscles, and the cervical vertebrae.

In 2015, I gave a lecture to the American Academy of gnathological orthopedists, in Phoenix. At the lecture, I presented a theory of how a bad bite can contribute to an unwarranted cervical cartilage operation. I feel that this medical problem needs more research and serious changes in the treatment of neck surgery.

The problem starts with a person's bad bite, which creates a temporal mandibular dysfunction. Three maxillary malpositions can create a temporal mandibular dysfunction, not counting accidents. I would like to refer the three positions to a pilot's jargon. An over closed bite {often caused by developing a resting tongue position (tongue splinting) when young}, causes a "pitch" or forward head position. The head weighs about 12 to 14 pounds. When the head is postured forward, it changes the posture, causing scoliosis of the cervical spine. This position, according to Dr. Janet Travell, creates posterior neck muscle tension. This is often exhibited by posterior neck tension and headaches. Two other positions also create neck tension, but not on the posterior of the vertebrae. They are a canted (class IV bite), "roll", and an atlas/axis malposition, "yaw." The neck muscle tension for these malocclusions is not directly from the posterior, which is present with an over closed bite. However, a canted bite can cause neck tension that also can change the vertebral posture and scoliosis.

When the over closed temporal mandibular dysfunction patient's forward posture creates scoliosis, it affects vertebral cartilages C2, C3, C4, C5, and C6. It affects the anterior portion of the vertebrae, which puts undue pressure on the anterior part of the cervical cartilages, between the vertebrae.

Many dentists do not relate a TMJ dysfunction problem with the blood pH and cervical vertebrae. But now another factor comes into play, an acidic body, the body cell and blood pH, and the heart rhythm. With a very acidic body, or with a calcium deficiency, the calcium is usually deficient, and the pH of the blood can get below 7.4.

The heart rhythm depends on a constant blood pH of 7.4, to keep a steady pace. A lowering of the pH can cause the heart rhythm to slow down. But this is protected by the chemicals in the blood. They call out for calcium to raise the blood pH.

With a lowering of the blood pH, the chemicals in the blood seek calcium from the body to maintain a steady heart rhythm. If the calcium levels are not raised, this can also cause other heart problems.

Where does this calcium come from? It comes from bone areas that are under infection, tension, pressure, or stress. These conditions create osteoclasts. Osteoclasts gather and distribute the bone particles into the blood, to raise the pH to 7.4. The calcium can come from the periodontal bone between the teeth, and/or the anterior portion of the vertebral cartilages, under pressure from the forward head posture, caused by the scoliosis. The anterior cartilages, then, get degenerated, from the loss of calcium. Neck surgeons then surgically replace the cartilages.

Most dentists, oral surgeons, neck surgeons, and chiropractors do not relate the posture and anterior vertebral cervical cartilage degeneration, to 1. the over closed bite, 2. the TMJ dysfunction, 3. forward head posture, 4. posterior neck muscle tension, 5. anterior cervical vertebral scoliosis, 6. pressure on the anterior of the vertebral neck cartilages. 7. acidic blood pH, below 7.4, 8. calcium deficiency, and 9. slowed heart rhythm. These factors are all related to this complicated paradox. A person needs to know the sequence, to understand the serious problem. More research and study needs to be done, to understand the complicated biochemistry and surgical ramifications.

HUNDREDS of anterior cervical cartilage operations are done by neck surgeons every year that are caused by this acidic diet, LOW BLOOD pH, anterior vertebral scoliosis, anterior cartilage degeneration paradox. The neck surgeons, oral surgeons, dentists, and also chiropractors do not realize that the acidic blood pH, the over closed bite, TMJ dysfunction, forward head posture, anterior scoliosis, and anterior cervical vertebral cartilage degeneration, is the cause of the problem. The neck surgery all starts with the TMJ dysfunction and the forward anterior head posture.

Dentists and other professionals need to understand the importance of an acidic body, and how an acetic diet, body cells, the blood pH, calcium deficiency, and cervical vertebral cartilage degeneration are related to their professions.

Now, I would like to ask another question. If there is scoliosis of the vertebral vertebrae, does it relate to scoliosis of the lumbar vertebrae? If it does, then the iliopsoas muscle attaches from the lower lumbar vertebrae through the pelvis to the femur. Would that distortion be the cause of a short leg?

38

Four-In-One Onnetsu Therapy

(With Permission from Budwig Cancer Clinic)

The text in the following chapter has been given to the Budwig Cancer Clinic patients.

Ancient Japanese and oriental medicine consider cancer as a 'cold' disease and applying just the right amount of heat for specific periods of time can produce outstanding results.

"Those who cannot be cured by medicine may be cured by surgery. Those who cannot be cured by surgery may be cured by heat. Those who cannot be cured by heat are to be considered incurable."

—Hippocrates (460 BC – 370 BC)

From this concept is born a therapy in the early part of the year 2000 that combines (1) heat, (2) acupuncture (but without the needles), (3) energy balancing and (4) vibrational frequencies all in one, called "Four in One" therapy.

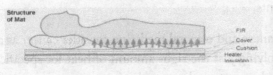

Four-In-One Therapy

4 Therapies administered simultaneously with
a special Mat and/or Handheld wand

Far Infrared Therapy

Electro Magnetic Frequencies

Volcanic Minerals

Acupuncture Therapy

Cancer cell

Warm ⇕ **Cold**

Unhealthy Cold Cells

Structure of Mat

FIR
Cover
Cushion
Heater
Insulation

Using four effective therapies, simultaneously, all combined into one is a breakthrough in cancer treatment as can be seen from these clinical studies:

CLINICAL STUDIES

STUDY CASE A: BREAST CANCER CASE STORY

On June 25, 2018. The person (Female, Age 69) came, being rejected by hospitals as "Incurable".

• Breast cancer patient was given only 2 or 3 days to live from her Oncologist

• Size of breast tumor was 15cm (6 inches) about size of a melon

• Tumor was extending from breast and had a very foul smell

• Four in One Hand Wand therapy applied on her spinal column daily

• Lymphocytes began increasing in about 14 days and condition improved

• 2 weeks into program the tumor fell off the breast

• Slept on Four in One Blanket on "High or 5 = 48°C" for 30 minutes then reduce the heat to 1=38°C or 2.

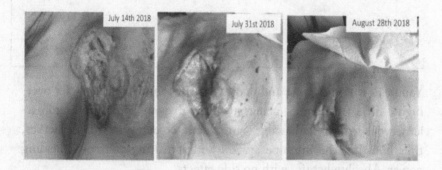

STUDY CASE B - STAGE 4 MELANOMA PATIENT (MALE)

• Four-In-One therapy began in June 12, 2013

• 3 weeks of daily spinal treatment and sleeping on Four in One blanket

• 3 weeks later Melanoma great improved and in 2018 still doing very well

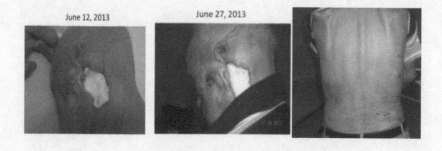

Dr. Johanna Budwig was constantly talking about the benefits of sunlight and natural heat. Now as time goes on more and more scientists are finding how she was ahead of her time in this research. The Onnetsu Mattress offers all FOUR-IN-ONE therapies simultaneously while you sleep at night.

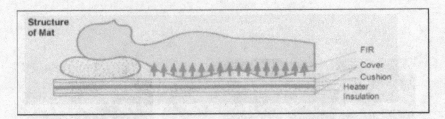

You lie down on the mat and make yourself comfortable, even for overnight. The frequencies penetrate through your spine into automatic nervous system, balancing sympathetic & parasympathetic nerves, thus boosting the immune system and activating your own healing power. Absolutely safe, with no side effects.

This is nothing like a heating pad or electric blanket. The thermostat control is very precise, prevents overheating and always maintains a comfortable temperature. High, Med, Low. The control system does not allow any harmful EMF frequencies to reach the body.

Works on both 100-240V - Size: 21⊠ x 52⊠ inches (53 x 132 cm)

Vinyl leather cover is very sanitary and safe even if you spill water on it. Clean with wet towels only. You put a cotton sheet over the mat and can also be used to steam heat the body by using wet towels.

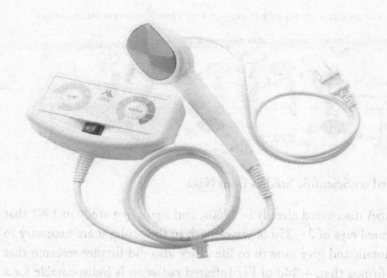

FOUR IN ONE HEALING WAND

This device is designed to pass over the entire spinal column. Every organ in the body is represented in the spinal column. When a person notices a slight "ouch" this is a sign that area needs therapy. Also, the healing wand is passed over all areas of the body that are ill and need attention. This activates the bodies natural healing mode.

This FOUR IN ONE Thermotherapy revives the function of Autonomic Nervous Systems by balancing the Sympathetic and Parasympathetic nerves, promotes circulations of blood, hormone balancing. It improves the immune system at the same time. It is completely natural and harmless. There is no side effect.

Videos are provided to all patients so they can understand and see how the FOUR IN ONE healing wand is used.

Therapists at the Budwig Center will administer a 45-minute session every day on each patient.

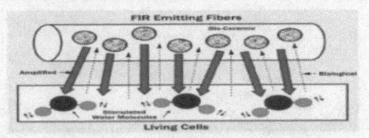

Based on Scientific Studies from Nasa

NASA discovered already in 1960s, and again in a study in 1981 that infrared rays of 2 – 25μ of wavelength in the sunlight are necessary to maintain and give growth to life. They also did further research that confirmed that, 4~14μ of Far Infrared radiation is indispensable for a living body's metabolism, rejuvenation, healing, growth, upbringing, making heat energy to occur by a resonance action with cell molecules in a human body.

Raymond Rife in 1920s-30s used this theory to produce a machine to destroy microorganisms with resonant frequency or vibration called a frequency generator.

How the Four-In-One Therapy Works

(1) Acupuncture (without the needles)

Acupuncture stimulates certain points on the body, most often with a needle penetrating the skin and probably excites the biochemical responses in the human body via the nerves, thus releasing feel-good chemicals that can aid in inflammation, stress, and so forth.

The Four-In-One therapy capitalizes on this acupuncture methodology to deliver heat and selected frequencies to the affected areas, thus greatly speeding up the process of reversing the cancer.

[2] Hyperthermia

Hyperthermia creates heat and initiates a fever-like state, causing an intense, sustained elevation in core body temperature, which enhances the immune system and therefore activates a natural self-healing process in the body.

"In July 2013, The Lancet Oncology published an article on the beneficial effects of hyperthermia (heat therapy). A team of clinicians headed by Rüdiger Wessalowski, MD of the University of Düsseldorf, showed that conventional treatment that included deep-tissue heating produced better results than generally achieved with surgery, radiation and/or chemotherapy alone.

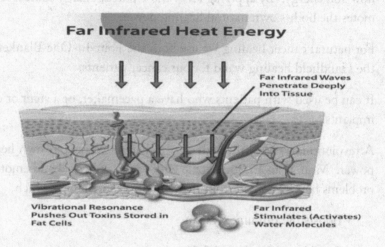

Far Infrared light therapy penetrates deep into the tissues

(3) Vibrational Frequencies

Dr. Royal Rife, Dr. Hulda Clark and Dr. Bob Beck proved that it is possible to destroy cancer causing viruses by bombarding them with selected frequencies. Using volcano rocks from the Aso Mountain of Japan the Four-In-One therapy sends a vibration to the affected areas. Four-In-One therapy creates a wave vibration that can activate cells deep in the body and can create an environment where abnormal cells (malignant tumor etc.) cannot live.

With the combination of Far-Infrared ray and the volcanic rock, these waves begin resonating into cells with great speed and incredible precision to penetrate cancer cells.

(4) Balance

In Chinese medicine when the "cold" and "hot" spots (they call yin and yang) are out of balance this produces disease. The Four-In-One handheld wand and/or blanket detects the "cold" spots of the body and brings them into balance.

The Four-In-One therapy is completely harmless and non-invasive as it provides vibrations, heat, balance and increased blood and lymphatic flow and energy. By applying all of these potent energy sources it promotes the body's own natural healing power.

For natural cancer healing we use both the Four-In-One Blanket and the Handheld healing wand for our cancer patients.

It can be used with patients who have a pacemaker, or a stent or other implants.

A revolutionary, breakthrough device that activates your own healing power. More than 15,000 people with various physical and emotional problems have benefited from the Four-In-One Therapy which:

- Boosts the Immune System

- Provides FIR infrared 5-20 microns wavelength (the same as the KI emitted by the human body and like the sun which is essential for every living cell

- Penetrates deeply into the body, corrects hormone imbalances

- Stimulates blood circulation

- Helps with Pain, fatigue and stress

- Improved organ functions

- Rejuvenates cells and repairs degenerated cells

- Facilitates elimination

- Helps with cancer as well as many common diseases such as: Arthritis, asthma, bladder, blood pressure, abnormalities of

172

bones, various cancers, cold, diabetes, digestive problems, dizziness, fibroid, hepatitis, kidney and liver problems, lime disease, parasites, Parkinson's, stroke, thyroid problems, stress, various women's issues, abdominalgia, atopic dermatitis, autonomic imbalance, bladder, blood pressure, bipolar disorder, brain infarction, brain tumor, abnormalities of bones, adhesive capsulitis of shoulder, cold, cardiac arrhythmia, cataract, cerebral thrombus, Charley horse, chronic leukemia, colitis, contracted kidney, duodenal ulcer, diabetes, digestive problems, dizziness, dyspnea, eye and ear problems, fibroid, Graves-Basedow disease, gastric ulcer, headache, heartburn, hepatitis, hemorrhoid, herniated disc, herpes zoster, HIV, infertility, insomnia, intercostal neuralgia, kidney and liver problems, lime disease, low back pain, lymphedema, Ménière's disease, migraine headache, night urination, parasites, palpitation, Parkinson's disease, pollen allergy, protein in urine, reflux esophagitis, rheumatism, rhinitis, stroke, sciatic pain, shortness of breath, spine injury, strained eye, thyroid problems, tinnitus, trigeminal neuralgia, Tuberculosis, tinnitus, trigeminal neuralgia, Tuberculosis, thromboangiitis obliterans, ulcerative colitis, urocystitis, cystitis, vomiting, whiplash injury, xerophthalmia, yellow ligament, vomiting, whiplash injury, problem by helping promotion of one's own healing power.

39

Summary and Rx Schedule
for 23 Cancer Treatments

In many foreign countries, many cancer physicians have had an 85 to 90 percent cure rate treating over 200,000 cancer patients. The following summary of the 22 treatments is very important and is used by physicians all over the world to cure cancer. Even if you use the four customary treatments used by oncologists, these treatments will help you. They are non-invasive.

These 22 summaries will help you and your cancer manager, find where to obtain these supplements, foods, minerals, and treatments. It will explain how to use the things needed and time schedules. Please check the dosages with your physician, to be sure they are correct. Refrain from using any treatments which create allergic or unforeseen problems.

Treatment 1: Joanna Budwig's cottage cheese, quark, flaxseed oil Tx.

The double helix bond treatment is used for unraveling sticky blood, present in 80-90 percent of cancer patients. This treatment is fully explained in chapter one of this book. I consider it to be the NUMBER ONE PROCEDURE for stopping and helping cure cancer, for every patient, whether they are getting conventional chemo and radiation treatment, or alternative cancer treatment.

Treatment 2: Pancreatic enzymes.

Many enzymes are needed to digest dead cancer, debris, and protein particles in the blood, and at the cancer tumor site.

They are CRITICAL and essential every day. With cancer, 15 to 18 each day between meals.

1. Solozymes from www.collegehealthstores.com, or by calling 817 458 9241.

2. Wobenzym-N enzymes can be obtained at Amazon.com or on a computer. Their address is Garden of Life, 5,000 Village Blvd., West Palm Beach, Fl. 33407. With cancer, 15 to 18 enzymes are needed each day between meals.

Treatment 3: Sugar:

STOP ALL SUGARS, sugar products, vegetable oils gotten from the grocery shelf, fried and deep-fried foods, refined and processed foods, and RED meat, including beef and pork. These are cancer foods that cause sticky blood. Cancer cells love protein.

Treatment 4: Live electromagnetic foods.

What to eat: Two to three glasses of raw, fresh vegetable juices every day, with lemon, or 8 to 12 raw fresh vegetables in salads, twice daily. Three to four raw nuts, almonds, pecans, and walnuts, to provide the protein and oils needed each day. Fermented foods, fresh raw berries, squash, bulbs, roots, and leaves.

Treatment 5: GMO Foods.

Avoid all GMO foods: BUY ORGANIC. Do not eat any sugar beets, soy, or corn products. Avoid all breakfast cereals, bread, flour products.

Treatment 6: Coffee Enemas.

Coffee enemas: Coffee enemas are a very critical and essential practice, every day. Your cancer manager can help you with this. Your body cannot get rid of all the massive dead body cells, dead cancer cells, wastes, protein, and food particles in the blood. The liver and gall bladder need help detoxifying everything. Do not skip this procedure. Obtain a Gerson enema kit at Amazon.com.

Treatment 7: Barley Powder.

Barley powder: This is a very critical cancer alkaline food, gotten in flour form, or capsules. Many capsules are needed if your pH is acidic. You need to get hydrion litmus paper to find the acid/base reading or pH. 4.5 to 9 pH, litmus paper gotten can be obtained from Micro Essential Laboratory, Inc., 4224 Avenue H, Brooklyn, New York, 11201, or from Daily manufacturing, 800 868 0700, or at many health food stores. You can use the powder in soups and other foods. It may take as many as 12 to 15 Barley capsules to raise your pH to neutral (6.4). Barley powder can be bought at health food stores. Barley capsules can be obtained from "Green Supreme." 800 358 0777, or www.GreenSupreme. net

Treatment 8: Supplements.

Oral vitamin C, L-proline, and L-lysine. With cancer, do not skip this combination treatment. These kill cancer in its tracks. A combination of these capsules can be gotten from www.MakingHealthAffordable. com, They are called "Heart Plus." With cancer, take 6 tablets a day, between meals.

Treatment 9: Beta 3D Glucan.

Beta 3D glucan; An immune system booster that works in the blood.

You can obtain it by calling 855 877 8220, or by the website; www. ancient5.com

Treatment 10:

Raw, Fresh Vegetable Juice. Raw, fresh vegetable juice: If your cancer manager will help you, 3 to 4 glasses of raw fresh vegetable juice with lemons, is one of the best cancer treatments, every day. The Gerson cancer clinic gives their cancer patients 4 to 5 glasses of raw fresh vegetable juice every day. They use about 20 lbs. of raw, fresh vegetables per person. Even if you make one or two glasses, it will be a great help to cure cancer.

Treatment 11: Acidic Red Meat.

Red meat: With cancer, eat no red meat, beef, or pork. Limit white meat to two to three times a week. Eat raw nuts to give you protein. Almonds, walnuts, pecans, apricot seeds, and pistachios are very good protein foods.

Treatment 12: Fenbendazole.

Fenbendazole: cures cancer. Ask Joe Tippens. He used fenbendazole, (trade name "Panacur)" to cure his cancer (see chapter 16). This is a parasite cleanser and is great for eliminating parasites also, which is one of the things needed when a person has cancer. Joe used fenbendazole with three other supplements, vitamin E succinate, turmeric, and CBD oil (cannabinoid oil). A person can get fenbendazole at www. thelifetree.com. It is called; "purify."

Treatment 13: Nitric Oxide Supplements = Oxygen

Vitamin D3, turmeric, resveratrol, Ginkgo Biloba, L-arginine, L-theanine, and L-citrulline. When you have cancer, it is wise to take Vitamin D3, 25,000 IU for at least two months, then reduce the dosage to 10,000 IU. Take 2 tablets of turmeric, take 2 tablets of ginkgo Biloba, 200 mg L-arginine, 200 mg L-theanine, and 200 mg of L-citrulline. The tablets can be gotten at the health food store, or online. These supplements provide nitric oxide, which converts to oxygen in the body, vitally needed for cancer treatment.

Treatment 14: Root Canals

Root canals. With cancer, it is recommended to remove root canal teeth, because most older root canals are not sterile, and leak bacteria into the blood. It is said that newer root canals are more sterile.

Treatment 15: Insula Peptide

Insula peptide. Peptides are formed from amino acids. They are related to enzymes and are very vital for treating cancer. In Mexico, many cancer physicians use peptides, both I.V. and orally. They are very effective for curing cancer. You can get peptides from New England Peptides, 1 800 343 5974, or on the internet, sales@newenglandpeptide.com You will need to talk to a representative to find out which dosage is best for you.

Treatment 16: Dr. Joanna Budwig's Cancer Clinic

Dr. Joanna Budwig's cancer clinic. One of the best cancer clinics in the world is located near Malaga, Spain. If you have cancer and have the finances to go to Spain, then the Budwig clinic has the most updated procedures you could find that cure cancer. Dr. Budwig, a biochemist, started the clinic many years ago. They have been increasing their cancer cure rate ever since. They have many therapies, and their cure rate for cancer is way above average.

Treatment 17: Hyperthermia.

Hyperthermia. The infra-red sauna, and/or hot baths should be on your schedule every day when you have cancer. Cancer cells are suppressed, weakened, and knocked down when people can raise their body temperature over 102 degrees Fahrenheit. High heat also improves blood circulation and helps remove toxins. At Dr. Budwig's cancer clinic in Spain, every cancer patient is required to have a hyperthermia 4 in 1 treatment every day.

Treatment 18: Apricot Seeds, Laetrile.

Apricot seeds, and laetrile. In Mexico, many cancer physicians use laetrile and/or apricot seeds to help cure cancer. Other cancer physicians prescribe 10 to 15 apricot seeds a day. They are very successful in helping to cure cancer. They are a great cancer cell destroyer. Apricot seeds can be obtained from "Lucky Vitamin," 1-888-635-0474, and/or "Apricot Seeds." 1-800-383-6008. Laetrile can be obtained at a Mexican pharmacy by calling 1-888-271-4184.

Treatment 19: Mercury Fillings.

Mercury fillings, Amalgam fillings contain about 50 percent mercury. With cancer, since mercury is a poison, many alternative cancer physicians are recommending that cancer patients have their mercury fillings removed. It needs to be done by a dentist who is trained in amalgam removal.

Treatment 20: Hydrion Litmus Paper.

pH testing with Hydrion litmus paper. This is badly needed by every cancer patient. Take the pH of saliva and urine every night before brushing your teeth, and every morning when you get up. Buy the range between 4.5 and 8 or 9 pH. If it is not available at a health food store, you can order it from Daily Manufacturing, 1 800 782 7326, or Micro Essential Laboratory,

Inc., 4224 Avenue H, Brooklyn, New York, 11201

Treatment 21: Microwaved Food.

Microwave use. The microwave nukes all food, leaving a dead non-electromagnetic (dead) food. It is best to use the oven for warming any food.

Treatment 22: Garlic

Raw, fresh fermented black garlic is very valuable when a person has cancer. It is a superfood. Four to five cloves of crushed or chopped garlic in food, is a great health treatment, every day. Fresh fermented black garlic capsules are also available at health food stores and Daily Manufacturing.

Treatment 23: 4 in 1 Therapy

The Four in One mattress is a new instrument that has been introduced by the Budwig clinic in Spain to treat cancer. It is a great addition to cancer treatment and has been a great help in curing cancer. You will be able to read about it in chapter 38. Hopefully, with FDA approval, it will be used in the U.S. soon, to help cure cancer.

Treatment 24: The CellSonic VIPP Therapy Machine.

Recently, a new cancer therapy machine was introduced to the world market. It is now being used in India, Spain, Germany, France, England, and many other countries. It helps cure cancer and many other diseases. You can read about its success in Chapter 12. It is waiting for FDA approval in the U.S

The treatments in the preceding pages are a summary of the treatments in the book. I have tried to list them as a way for any cancer patient and manager to easily find the treatments, dosages, plus where to obtain the many products needed to cure cancer. *NOTE*: If you have cancer, all of these products, supplements, and procedures are needed to cure your cancer. By not using all of these procedures, it may result in not curing your cancer.

These products may cost some money, but money is not nearly as important as your life. The cost is not only worth your life, but will be the most rewarding chapter in your life.

I want to emphasize again the use of a CANCER MANAGER to help you cure cancer. Without an assistant, many cancer patients fail to buy and use the necessary foods, supplements, minerals, procedures, and treatments that are needed to cure cancer.

There are two other important cautions. If you smoke, drink much alcohol, or are on drugs, cancer treatment will be a failure. Steve McQueen ended up a cancer victim because he would not stop his bad habits. The other most important thing is to have faith in God. With faith and this combination of treatments and procedures, you can beat cancer. Stress, worry, and negative thinking are very detrimental when you have cancer. Good luck, you will win, and God Bless.

40

The Universal Force

Most people have known the genius in Albert Einstein's famous relativity papers. There is one force that he had not made famous, but it is a force that should be known and used throughout the world. If every person in the world would understand and abide by this magnificent universal force, there would be no disputes or wars. There would be no rift between the liberals and the conservatives. It would conquer everything, transcend everything, and be the quintessence of life.

In the late 1980s, Lieseri, the daughter of the famous genius, donated 1,400 letters, written by Einstein, to the Hebrew University, with orders not to publish their contents until two decades after his death. Here is one of the letters, sent to Lieseri.

"... When I proposed the theory of relativity, very few understood me, and what I will reveal now to transmit to mankind will also collide with the misunderstanding and prejudice in the world.

I ask you to guard the letters as long as necessary, years, decades until society is advanced enough to accept what I will explain below. There is an extremely powerful force that, so far, science has not found a formal explanation. It is a force that includes and governs all others, and is even behind any phenomenon operating in the universe, and has not yet been completely identified by us.

This universal force is love. When scientists looked for a unified theory of the universe, they forgot the most powerful unseen force. Love is Light, which enlightens those who give and receive it. Love is Gravity because it makes some people attracted to others. Love is power, because it multiplies the best we have, and allows humanity not to be extinguished in their blind selfish-

ness. Love unfolds and reveals. For love, we live and die. Love is god, and God is love.

This force explains everything and gives meaning to life. This is the variable that we have ignored for too long, maybe because we are afraid of love because it is the only energy in the universe that man has not learned to drive at will.

To give visibility to love I made a simple substitution in my most famous equation. If instead of $E = mc2$, we accept that the energy to heal the world can be obtained through love multiplied by the speed of light squared, we arrive at the conclusion that love is the most powerful force there is, because it has no limits.

After the failure of humanity in the use and control of the other forces of the universe that have turned against us, it is urgent that we nourish ourselves with another kind of energy.

If we want our species to survive, if we are to find meaning to live, if we want to save the world and every sentient being that inhabits it, love is the only answer.

Perhaps we are not yet ready to make a bomb of love, a device powerful enough to destroy the hate, selfishness, and greed that devastates the planet.

However, each individual carries within them a small but powerful generator of love whose energy is waiting to be released.

When we learn to give and receive this universal energy, dear Lieseri, we will have affirmed that love conquers all, is able to transcend everything and anything, because love is the quintessence of life.

I deeply regret not having been able to express what is in my heart, which has quietly beaten for you all of my life. Maybe it's too late to apologize, but as time is relative, I need to tell you that I love you, and thanks to you, I have reached the ultimate answer.

—*Your father, Albert Einstein*"

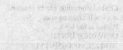

CPSIA information can be obtained
at www.ICGtesting.com
Printed in the USA
LVHW030024301221
707422LV00005B/151

9 781952 685088